Effective Supervisory Relationships

Effective Supervisory Relationships

Best Evidence and Practice

Helen Beinart and Sue Clohessy

WILEY Blackwell

Registered Offices
John Wiley & Sons, Inc., 111 River Street, Hoboken, NJ 07030, USA
John Wiley & Sons Ltd, The Atrium, Southern Gate, Chichester, West Sussex, PO19 8SQ, UK

Editorial Office
The Atrium, Southern Gate, Chichester, West Sussex, PO19 8SQ, UK

For details of our global editorial offices, customer services, and more information about Wiley products visit us at www.wiley.com.

Wiley also publishes its books in a variety of electronic formats and by print-on-demand. Some content that appears in standard print versions of this book may not be available in other formats.

Library of Congress Cataloging-in-Publication Data

Names: Beinart, Helen, author. | Clohessy, Sue, 1969– author.
Title: Effective supervisory relationships : best evidence and practice / Helen Beinart, Sue Clohessy.
Description: Hoboken : Wiley-Blackwell, 2017. | Includes bibliographical references and index.
Identifiers: LCCN 2016059296 (print) | LCCN 2017007815 (ebook) |
    ISBN 9781118973639 (hardback) | ISBN 9781118973622 (paper) |
    ISBN 9781118973615 (pdf) | ISBN 9781118973608 (epub)
Subjects: LCSH: Supervision. | Leadership–Psychological aspects. | Clinical psychology. |
    BISAC: PSYCHOLOGY / Clinical Psychology.
Classification: LCC HM1253 .B45 2017 (print) | LCC HM1253 (ebook) | DDC 303.3/4–dc23
LC record available at https://lccn.loc.gov/2016059296

Cover design: Wiley
Cover image: © Jasmina007/Getty Images

Set in 10/12pt Warnock by SPi Global, Pondicherry, India

Contents

About the Authors

Dr Helen Beinart works freelance as a supervisor and trainer, and as a Tutor on the Post-Graduate Certificate in Supervision at the University of Oxford. Previously she was Director (Clinical and Professional) of the Oxford Institute of Clinical Psychology Training, Oxford University (1994–2013). Clinically, she worked with children, young people, and their families in health and primary care settings. She trained in Cape Town and London and qualified as a clinical psychologist from the Institute of Psychiatry in 1979. She worked in the National Health Service for 40 years as a clinician, service manager, consultant, supervisor, and trainer. Since the mid-1990s, she has been involved in clinical psychology training, supervisor training, and research into the supervisory relationship. Prior to this she was Head of Child and Adolescent Health Clinical Psychology Services in Aylesbury and Kingston. She has chaired the Division of Clinical Psychology's Faculty for Children and Young People, and was involved in providing psychological evidence to the Parliamentary Select Committee on Children's Mental Health. Professionally she has held several roles within clinical psychology and has acted as national assessor for senior appointments to the profession, external examiner, adviser, supervisor, and teacher to a number of courses and services. She is author of several chapters and papers on clinical supervision and co-editor of *Clinical Psychology in Practice* (2009), together with Paul Kennedy and Sue Llewelyn. She has a long-term interest in the development of professional competence and the contribution of clinical supervision and, in particular, supervisory relationships to the development of competent practitioners.

Dr Sue Clohessy is Course Director of the Post-Graduate Certificate in Supervision of Applied Psychological Practice, Clinical Tutor, and the lead for supervisor training at the Oxford Institute of Clinical Psychology Training, University of Oxford. She completed her clinical training on the Oxford course in 1995, and since then has worked clinically in the field of adult mental health and trauma in NHS services in Buckinghamshire, Berkshire, and Oxfordshire in the United Kingdom. She now works clinically in independent practice and offers supervision to counsellors, psychologists, and CBT (cognitive behavioral therapy) practitioners. She completed the Diploma in Cognitive Therapy at the Oxford Cognitive Therapy Centre (OCTC), Warneford Hospital, in 2000, and is an Associate of OCTC, having been involved in supervising and examining academic submissions for their courses and having chaired the Board of Examiners for their advanced diploma and MSc courses. She is accredited as a CBT practitioner and supervisor with the British Association of Behavioural and Cognitive Psychotherapies (BABCP). She completed a post-qualification doctorate in the area of supervision and the supervisory relationship in 2008. She regularly teaches a range of professionals on supervision skills and has developed an Introduction to Clinical Supervision course for local supervisors based on national learning outcomes. She has worked with others in the clinical psychology training community on the development of national learning outcomes for advanced supervisor training, and is part of the Clinical Supervision Advisory Group. She has co-authored chapters and papers on supervision, and has contributed to the development of measures of the supervisory relationship and supervision competence.

Preface

Supervisees who have worked with us will be familiar with the phrase "Some supervisees' worst experiences with a supervisor may be another person's best experience" and vice versa. This reflects our belief that the quality of the supervisory relationship (SR) is pivotal to any experience of supervision and is unique to the individuals involved. It is the idiosyncratic matching of needs, learning styles, attitudes, and values that influences the experience. For example, an independent supervisee who is used to working autonomously is likely to find a supervisory relationship with a supervisor with exacting standards and a tendency to be directive in their supervision oppressive, and may feel resentful and devalued. However, a more anxious or perfectionistic supervisee may find their SR with a supervisor who expresses clear goals and requirements and has a directive approach containing and supportive. A good supervisor, therefore, needs to be flexible enough to adjust their style for each supervisee and, of course, not all people can do this. It may, therefore, be that lack of attention to the particular needs of the supervisee and lack of flexibility are more of a problem for SRs than any particular or preferred style.

Our thoughts in this area have developed from experiencing and working with multiple SRs. Helen Beinart, in her clinical role working with children, young people, and families, supervised trainee clinical psychologists from a number of UK training programs. As she became more senior, she also supervised qualified staff from a range of professional groups. At that time, in the National Health Service's (NHS) psychological services for children clinical, professional, and managerial supervisory roles were often conflated and the different tasks and functions of supervision needed to be clarified to effectively manage these SRs. During this period, HB became curious about the role of power and culture within the SR and noted how different supervisees needed and encouraged different emphases within their SRs. Sue Clohessy has worked clinically in adult mental health services throughout her career, and has been involved in supervising trainee psychologists and other professionals. Although there were differences in these supervision experiences, in particular relating to the expectations and the meaning of supervision for different professional groups, there were also many similarities. SC was struck by the wealth of training opportunities for developing clinical and therapeutic skills and the comparatively limited training in the skills needed to be a good supervisor. As such, she did what many supervisors have done and tried to emulate the good supervisors and the effective SRs that she had experienced.

A substantive part of both our careers has been in training roles within the Doctorate of Clinical Psychology (DClinPsych) program at Oxford, and as such our involvement in SRs has changed over the years. SC is currently a clinical tutor on the program, and HB was one of the course directors until she retired recently. The tutor role involves supporting and monitoring clinical placements, predominantly within NHS services. Supervisees normally work with one or two supervisors for a six-month period in the context of a range of different populations (e.g., adults, children, those who are learning-disabled, and the elderly) and clinical services (e.g., mental health, pediatric, neurodisability). Some SRs work very well and others less so, and the role of the tutor is to support and advise these SRs. Additionally, HB's role as course director involved multiple supervisor and line management responsibilities, a complex set of tasks and functions, together with shifting power relationships that had to be negotiated and managed. Our experiences in training have offered us the privilege of working with many different SRs and of developing a bird's-eye view of how the dyads work more or less effectively. This has contributed to our curiosity about the relational "ingredients" needed to make SRs successful. Our roles have involved listening to different perspectives (both supervisor and supervisee) on the SR and facilitating conversations about any difficulties that may be experienced by one or both parties. This has offered a perspective on SRs that has been enriched by multiple points of view and has led to an appreciation that dyads are unique, that supervisee needs will change, and that SRs work best when there is investment and flexibility on both sides. It has led to an appreciation of the power and influence of these relationships. At their best they can be inspiring and rewarding and can shape the professional self. When they are difficult, they can be frustrating, upsetting, damaging to self-confidence, and difficult to leave behind, their influence often felt in future SRs.

In addition to experiencing and witnessing many SRs from the outside, we have of course also been in SRs ourselves over our career pathways and, as supervisees, have found some more supportive, challenging, and conducive to learning and others less so. Additionally we have had an SR ourselves, which has had many guises including clinical, professional, research, and managerial supervision. We reflect on our own SR in the Endnote of this book and apply some of the material that we cover to exemplify how the supervision literature can be applied.

Our research interests developed from witnessing many successful, and some less successful, SRs. In particular, we became curious about the qualities of those SRs that worked more effectively than others. At this time (in the late 1990s), there was very little UK research on supervision and precious little on the SR but there were some interesting findings from the United States that pointed toward the SR being significant in supervision outcomes. There was also increasing recognition of the need to develop some more robust measures of the SR so that findings from any research that was undertaken could be more reliable and valid. Both of us have undertaken direct research into the quality of the SR, HB exploring the topic from a supervisee's perspective and SC from the perspective of the supervisor. Our role on the DClinPsych program has meant that we have been fortunate to have talented doctoral students interested in collaborating in this research. To date, eight doctoral dissertations have been undertaken as part of our research group. Three of these studies have worked on developing published measures that have recently been highlighted as a gold standard in supervision measures. Other studies have explored the development of the SR, self-disclosure, and how supervisees and supervisors manage difficulties within the SR (see www.oxcipt.co.uk for further details). Conducting research has also given us exposure to a different type of SR, from the perspective of both supervisee and supervisor and of research supervision. It has slowly dawned on us that the qualities inherent in effective and less effective SRs are evident in a range of different supervisory relationships, and that some of our findings (possibly with some adaptation) are applicable to a whole spectrum of different contexts.

Our experience of supporting numerous SRs, as well as our research in this area have also contributed to our enthusiasm for training others in key supervision skills, including the skills needed to establish and maintain effective supervisory relationships. We have benefited from working with our colleagues from other training programs who share a commitment to improving the quality of supervisor training and keeping supervision on the agenda in our profession. We have been involved with several national groups including Supervisor Training and Recognition, (STAR) and, later, the Clinical Supervision Advisory Group (CSAG). Our most exciting recent development, apart from writing this book, is running an Oxford University Postgraduate Certificate in Supervision for a range of professional groups. We have welcomed supervisors from clinical and applied psychology, nursing, education, psychotherapy, counseling, music therapy, and coaching, and we have mutually benefited from a rich learning environment in which we have explored the key skills needed for supervision, and how these can be applied in very different professional contexts.

We are fortunate that the research evidence to date supports our long-held beliefs that it is the quality of the SR that is the central factor in supervision. Hence, we think that it is important enough to write a book on the SR itself rather than a general book on supervision. We hope that you will find our material interesting and applicable. The book is divided into two sections: the first part focuses on research and theory and the second is more practice-oriented.

Acknowledgments

We would like to thank our colleagues at the Oxford Institute of Clinical Psychology Training for their interest and support in supervision over many years. We would particularly like to thank the Clinical Tutor team – Helen Jenkins, Kathryn Evans, David Dean, and Nigel King – with whom we have shared many supervision discussions. We would also like to thank our colleagues and Helen's co-directors of the institute at the time, Sue Llewelyn and Paul Kennedy, for their wisdom and support. We are particularly grateful to the late Paul Kennedy (1959–2016) for his help and encouragement during the recent development of the Post-Graduate Certificate in Supervision of Applied Psychological Practice.

We have found that working closely with trainee clinical psychologists and their supervisors supporting clinical placements has significantly contributed to our understanding of supervisory relationships. These are too numerous to thank by name but we would like to acknowledge their contribution to our learning, particularly those that posed some challenges!

We have been fortunate to attract talented doctoral trainees interested in research in supervision who have contributed significantly to our research program. We would like to thank Marina Palomo, Kate Frost, Nathalie Pearce, Clare Borsay, Vivien Lemoir, and Tom Cliffe for their interest, enthusiasm, and contribution to research on the supervisory relationship. Myra Cooper, Senior Research Tutor at the Institute, has made a significant contribution to this body of work and we have greatly valued her expertise and support.

The Oxford Institute has run residential supervisor training workshops on an annual basis over many years for our colleagues, supervisors, and trainees. We have benefited hugely through learning from many facilitators including Annie Mitchell and Kay Hughes from the University of Plymouth, and Joyce Scaife from the University of Sheffield, to name but a few. Many, but not all, of the facilitators for our residential training workshops have been drawn from the national Group of Trainers in Clinical Psychology and we have greatly valued our collaboration with the Supervisor Training and Recognition Group and the Clinical Supervision Advisory Group (CSAG).

We have also learned a great deal from developing and delivering a range of teaching programs for both clinical psychology supervisors and a broad range of applied psychology and professional supervisors. We would particularly like to acknowledge what we have learned through working closely with the first two cohorts who attended the Institute's Postgraduate Certificate in Supervision of Applied Psychological Practice.

We would like to thank our own supervisors, those who influenced us in our formative years as well as current supervisors, who continue to share their wisdom, support, and "safe challenges."

Last but definitely not least, we would like to thank our families who have seen us through many ups and downs in life and in work, and during the preparation of this book.

Part I

Effective Supervisory Relationships

Best Evidence

1

Introduction

There are many books on supervision but very few that focus specifically on the supervisory relationship (SR). Best evidence to date suggests that the SR is the most significant aspect of supervision and that it contributes to improved practice, as well as supervisee efficacy, resilience, and well-being. This book will provide the theory, research, and practice to support our readers in developing effective SRs and, in so doing, improved practice in their field of training or work.

The aim of the book is to provide cutting edge information on the SR based on current research and practice. We hope that this book will be useful and accessible to a broad range of practitioners who employ and apply psychological principles in their work, including applied psychologists, psychological therapists, mental health nurses, counselors, psychotherapists, and all those who work in health and social care (the helping professions). We consider these principles to be applicable to a broad audience, including those working in education and in the voluntary and independent sectors. For example, the coaching profession is developing rapidly and is beginning to require supervision as part of its practice. Those working in this field may find some of the material presented here very applicable.

The majority of published research on supervision draws from counseling psychology and psychotherapy, and much of the research has been conducted with those training to become applied psychologists. This is unsurprising as supervision is a central aspect of clinical and counseling psychology trainings. Supervision is also the core of training in the psychotherapy, medical, nursing, and social work professions and is a requirement for post-qualification professional practice in the majority of the helping professions. Although much of the literature that we refer to in the book will relate to these professional groups, we believe that many of the principles outlined in the development of effective SRs will also apply to other groups, including those working in educational and academic contexts.

The unique aspect of this book is its review of the evidence, drawing out of the themes, and identification of methods to improve practice in a range of settings. The first part focuses on the evidence base, reviews models of supervision,

Effective Supervisory Relationships: Best Evidence and Practice, First Edition.
Helen Beinart and Sue Clohessy.
© 2017 John Wiley & Sons Ltd. Published 2017 by John Wiley & Sons Ltd.

discusses the supervisory dyad in some detail, explores measurement and supervision outcomes, and, finally, considers issues of ethics, diversity, and power in supervision. The second part explores best practice based on current theory and evidence, including practical techniques and methods to establish, develop, and maintain effective SRs. We discuss setting up SRs in a way that is likely to make them succeed, giving and receiving meaningful feedback, managing any difficulties that arise, and supporting reflective practice and ongoing learning and development. Additionally, we explore new directions in the future development of effective SRs including working with groups and on-line.

The overwhelming finding from the emerging international evidence base within the dyadic supervision literature is that the SR is pivotal. Not only is it the vehicle through which supervision takes place but it is also the mutative aspect of supervision. This is illustrated by the following quotations from experts in the field: "good supervision is about the relationship, not the specific theory or techniques used" (Ellis, 2010, p. 106); "the supervisor–supervisee alliance has increasingly emerged as a variable of pre-eminent importance in the conceptualization and conduct of supervision … it is widely embraced as the very heart and soul of supervision" (Watkins, 2014a, p. 19). In the latter paper, Watkins presents a challenge to the reader (and subsequent authors) when he asks if we really know what the SR is about. We hope that, by the end of this book, readers will have a clear understanding of the SR and its significance to supervision outcomes for both research and practice.

In this introductory chapter we shall discuss definitions of supervision and the SR, identify the key elements of the SR, and discuss some of the competency frameworks in this developing field.

Definitions

Before defining the SR, it is perhaps worth defining supervision itself. Proctor and Inskipp (1988, p. 4) provide a broad definition:

> Supervision is a working alliance between supervisor and worker/s in which the worker can reflect on herself in her working situation by giving account of her work and receiving feedback and where appropriate, guidance and appraisal. The object of this alliance is to maximize the competence of the worker in providing a helping service.

Proctor and Inskipp (1988) identify three broad purposes of supervision, which have been widely accepted:

- *normative*: monitoring the quality of professional services, evaluation, gatekeeping for particular professional groups;
- *formative*: focusing on the development of the supervisee and enhancing professional competence;
- *restorative*: supporting the supervisee to express, process, and reflect on their work.

Milne (2009) describes an empirical definition of supervision, drawn from previous definitions, that aims to specify and operationalize key relationships and tasks. He defines it as

> the formal provision, by approved supervisors, of a relationship based education and training that is work focused and which manages, supports, develops, and evaluates the work of colleague/s. It therefore differs from related activities, such as mentoring and therapy, by incorporating an evaluative component and being obligatory. The main methods that supervisors use are corrective feedback on the supervisees' performance, teaching and collaborative goal-setting. (Milne, 2009, p. 15)

Both of the above definitions of supervision place a clear emphasis on the SR; however, there are limited definitions of the SR itself within the literature. These will now be reviewed in more detail, followed by our own working definition of the SR.

Bordin (1983) developed a working alliance model, the supervisory working alliance (SWA), defined as a mutual agreement on the goals and tasks of supervision and the bonds that develop between the supervisor and supervisee. He described supervision as a "collaboration for change," which provides a developmental context for the supervisee, the supervisor, and their work. Bordin's definition has been widely applied and the SWA has been accepted across many modalities of supervision. As we shall see in Chapter 2, it has also received a fair amount of research support. However, as the SWA is a direct translation from his psychotherapy working alliance model (Bordin, 1979), it may not fully reflect the complexity of supervision and how the SR differs from a psychotherapy relationship. The SR may include a working alliance between supervisor and supervisee, but it is also likely to include additional relational, educational, and contextual aspects (Beinart, 2014).

Holloway (1995, pp. 41–42) provided a more detailed definition of the SR. "The relationship is a container of a dynamic process in which supervisor and supervisee negotiate a personal way of using a structure of power and involvement that accommodates the supervisee's progression of learning." The SR is seen as developing through phases (beginning, middle, and end), changing over time, and being organized through a supervision contract. Holloway's model is one of the few that addresses power within the SR and that positions the development of the SR as central to broad contextual factors (supervisee, supervisor, client, and institution) and to the tasks and functions of supervision. This model will be discussed in more detail in Chapter 2.

Bernard and Goodyear (2014, p. 64) define the SR as

> the supervision participants' attitudes and feelings towards each other and the way in which those attitudes and feelings are expressed. The supervision relationship, an eminently triadic affair, encompasses such variables as the supervision alliance, attachment style, supervisory style, parallel process and personality factors.

This definition shows a clear understanding of the breadth and complexity of the SR. However, it assumes a three-person interaction between client, therapist/supervisee, and supervisor that places it very much within a therapy context. It is clear that supervision is a dyadic interaction where there is mutual influence between supervisor and supervisee. The supervisee is pivotal in selecting the work that they present to the supervisor. This work may be about an individual client, in which case the interaction may be triadic. However, many supervision issues are much broader than one-to-one therapy and may include work with families, teams, and, indeed, whole organizations – there are multiple contextual factors that influence the SR and the room is often very crowded. Additionally, supervision content may include aspects of work that are not directly therapeutic, for example, teaching, research, managing conflict with other staff, and reflective personal/professional development of the supervisee. Interestingly, a recent paper on the SR (Tangen & Borders, 2016) suggests that the complexity of the SR makes it difficult to conceptualize clearly.

Our own working definition, based on our research on the unique qualities of the SR, is as follows:

> The SR is a collaborative, mutual working relationship, which supports and challenges the supervisee to learn and develop their professional practice. The relationship is developmental, needs-focused, open, and respectful. It is normally hierarchical and involves the negotiation of power. It has many functions including education, monitoring and/or evaluation, and support. The SR is influenced by multiple contextual factors including those contributed by the supervisory dyad (or group), the working context, and the wider sociocultural context. The relationship is bound by the ethics of safe practice, and acknowledges difference and diversity in order to allow the supervisee to safely disclose and explore their professional dilemmas. Key tasks in establishing and developing the relationship are contracting and feedback.

Why Is the Supervisory Relationship Important?

Interestingly, supervision research has lagged behind therapy research despite almost all therapy trials requiring supervision, at the very least, to ensure adherence to the agreed treatment protocols. The focus of research has, understandably, been on client outcomes in a range of different interventions offered (e.g., anxiety and cognitive behavioral therapy [CBT]). It has been assumed that supervision is necessary for effective treatments, but its contribution to clinical outcome has been difficult to measure, and there is currently only a small body of research. (e.g., Bambling, King, Raue, Schweitzer, & Lambert, 2006).

The importance of the supervisory alliance was noted nearly 50 years ago (Watkins, 2014a) but until recently there has not been solid enough evidence to support this. However, in recent years, best evidence points to the SR as the mutative factor in the development of effective supervision (Beinart, 2014;

Watkins, 2014a); in particular, the development of a safe and supportive relationship has been shown to facilitate supervisee learning and development in a number of areas (see Chapter 3 for further discussion). Our research has focused particularly on the unique aspects of the SR that contribute to effectiveness. We have begun to unpick the contributions of supervisee and supervisor to the SR and to understand the importance of context to this relationship. We have used both qualitative and quantitative research methods to identify what it is about the SR that makes it work well and less well. It has become clear over the years that we have been doing this research, alongside supporting multiple SRs (as tutors on a doctoral training program in clinical psychology) and working within our own SRs, that there are certain elements that must be in place for these rather unusual relationships to work well. Our teaching across multiple professional groups has additionally confirmed the importance of the SR as the most significant aspect of supervision regardless of level of experience, although it does appear to carry particular significance for novice professionals. In particular, unsafe or unhelpful SRs are carried in the memory long after the event and often influence new supervisors when they begin to take on supervisory roles.

Key Elements in Effective Supervisory Relationships

It is important to take a meta-perspective when establishing an SR in order to have a conversation about the sort of SR each party would like to establish. In essence, supervisees and supervisors are working toward a psychological contract (Rousseau, 1995) about how they wish to work together (see Chapter 6). This involves creating an environment where it is possible to share uncertainties about the work and risk disclosing mistakes in order to allow sharing and learning to take place. Our research suggests that it is particularly important to establish clear boundaries in order to develop the trust required for this level of self-disclosure. Collaboration between supervisee and supervisor is important in order to establish clarity about roles and expectations. Supervisees need to be empowered to identify their learning needs and to explore their preferences for learning. Another important key skill is the mutual exchange of feedback and exploration of feedback preferences (see Chapter 7). In recent years the supervision literature has stressed the importance of being alert to cultural diversity in any approach to supervision and of the significance of having conversations that welcome diversity within the SR (e.g., Falender, Shafranske, & Falicov, 2014). It is also essential to consider ethical practice and to provide opportunities to engage in ethical debate and decision-making within the SR (see Chapter 5). Ladany (2014) stresses that features of ineffectual supervision include failing to take into account of, and be sensitive to, cultural and ethical issues; boundary violations; inappropriate use of, or failure to use, models and measures of supervision; and the misuse of power. Models are discussed in detail in Chapter 2 and measurement in Chapter 4. Boundaries and power are so key to the SR that they will be referred to throughout this book; difficulties are discussed in Chapter 6.

Competencies and Frameworks

Since the mid-2000s or so, there has been a strong competency movement within clinical supervision and a call for supervision to be seen as a professional competence in its own right and not just as an adjunct to practice. There has been strong criticism, from established experts (e.g., Falender & Shafranske, 2014; Ladany, 2014), of the assumption that being an experienced and competent practitioner makes one an effective supervisor. There are now clear competency frameworks for supervisors that have been developed and accepted in several countries. For example, in the United Kingdom the British Psychological Society (BPS) has adopted a set of learning outcomes for initial supervisor training, which are now part of the requirement to join the Register of Applied Psychology Practice Supervisors, held by the BPS. Unfortunately, for a number of reasons, supervisor training and registration is not mandatory for psychologists in the United Kingdom, which leaves some concern about quality control. This is not the case for psychological practitioners trained via the Improving Access to Psychological Therapies (IAPT) program in the United Kingdom, who are required to receive supervision by trained supervisors (Turpin & Wheeler, 2011). A set of competencies for supervisors has been developed within this program. These include a set of generic and meta-competencies that cover all therapeutic modalities and specific competencies for a range of therapeutic modalities (e.g., CBT, systemic therapy) (Roth & Pilling, 2008). The argument presented in the IAPT guidance is that supervision is the key to providing safe, effective, evidenced-based practice to ensure treatment fidelity. Whether this then impacts client outcomes is still a research question that needs further attention (Watkins, 2014a) and the IAPT program is in a good position to address this issue with the detailed data that it collects on routine clinical practice and outcomes.

In the United States the competency movement has gathered momentum, which has led to the development of a competency cube (Rodolfa et al., 2005) – a three-dimensional model representing foundational (e.g., reflective practice, relationships, ethics) and functional competencies (e.g., assessment and intervention) over the phases of professional development. In particular, Falender and Shafranske (2007, p. 233) have written emphatically about the need to train and assess supervisors to meet a set of agreed competencies:

> Competency based supervision is an approach that explicitly identifies the knowledge, skills and values assembled to form each clinical competency and develop learning strategies and evaluation procedures to meet criterion referenced competence standards in keeping with evidenced based practices and requirements of local clinical settings.

The American Psychological Association (APA) has not uniformly embraced the mandatory training of supervisors in order to meet competence-based supervisor training, which is mandatory only in a handful of states in the United States. However, the APA has recently approved agreed guidelines for clinical supervision in health service psychology (APA, 2015), which is a promising development.

Australia has led the way by introducing a national program of mandatory supervisor training. In 2013 the Psychology Board of Australia (PsyBA) introduced new supervisor training requirements that apply to all psychologists who provide supervision for provisional registrants undertaking internships and higher degree placements. All supervisors are required to undertake PsyBA-approved training in order to become an approved supervisor. PsyBA-approved supervisor training entails at least 20 hours of training presented in three sequentially completed parts: (a) knowledge assessment; (b) face-to-face skills training; and (c) competency-based assessment and evaluation. A further six hours of approved training is required every five years to maintain knowledge and skills. Board-approved supervisors must demonstrate proficiency in the following competencies:

1) knowledge and understanding of the profession
2) knowledge of and skills in effective supervision practices
3) knowledge of and ability to develop and manage the supervisory alliance
4) ability to assess the psychological competencies of the supervisee
5) capacity to evaluate the supervisory process
6) awareness of and attention to the diversity of client groups, and
7) ability to address the legal and ethical considerations related to the professional practice of psychology. (Psychology Board of Australia, 2013, pp. 4–5)

All of the aforementioned supervisor competency statements, whether or not training is mandatory, stress the importance of the SR as a key competence in clinical supervision. The Clinical Supervision Advisory Group (CSAG), part of the Group of Trainers in Clinical Psychology of the BPS, has developed guidance for the training of advanced competencies for experienced supervisors. This guidance describes characteristics of experienced supervisors—the section on the development of the SR is quoted in full:

Develops effective supervisory relationships:

1) Facilitates a supportive, collaborative and open supervisory relationship, with clear boundaries creating a safe space, which enables disclosure by supervisee of any concerns. Takes a pro-active stance in managing the supervisory relationship (SR), identifies and approaches any strains early on.
2) Acknowledges/manages complex power differentials, values difference, and invites feedback on the SR.
3) Values relationships in the context of training, maintaining effective relationship with the training course as well as the supervisee.
4) Demonstrates commitment and actively invests in supervision and the supervisee.
5) Promotes supervisee to take ownership of supervision as an active participant, e.g. setting agendas, goals, and reviewing learning outcomes.
6) Skilled and able to process the demands of managing multiple roles (e.g. educative, managerial, evaluative, supportive).

7) Develops supervision contracts with supervisees, and is clear about roles and responsibilities in supervision and the limits of confidentiality.
8) Addresses and reflects on ethical, relational and boundary issues effectively when they arise in supervision.
9) Achieves balance between direction and encouraging autonomy that includes appropriate risk taking, and effectively contains supervisee emotional responses to the work.
10) Applies models of supervision, learning and consultation and uses these to formulate and manage challenges within the SR. (Beinart & Golding, 2015, p. 32).

Of course, there is always debate and sometimes disagreement on how to describe the complex process of supervision, and multiple theories and models describe the process. Despite the growth of the competency movement, some schools of psychology argue that supervision is more of an art than a science and that much of what happens in a supervision session is intuitive, creative, and dependent on the individual chemistry within the dyad at that moment. There is also an emerging school of thought that suggests that supervisors should use mindfulness or meditative techniques to provide a safe and containing space for the supervisee (Sarnat, 2010). Applied psychologists with more scientific leanings would probably subsume these processes under the label of meta-competencies. However, regardless of approach, and of the narrative informed by this approach, it remains incontrovertible that effective supervision takes place in the process that occurs between supervisor and supervisee, and that certain relational fundamentals need to be in place for this to occur. It is essential that we attempt to identify and define these competencies so that we can consistently educate and train effective supervisors and measure both process and outcomes achieved. This leads us on to discussing how other influences and different contexts may influence and shape the SR.

Contextual Influences

Much of the literature in clinical supervision stems from training contexts. There is more research reflecting the experiences of clinical and counseling psychologists in training than of those post-qualification. The participants in our research are all trainee clinical psychologists on accredited UK training courses and their clinical supervisors. The supervision competencies described earlier largely refer to the competencies required for pre-qualification training. The training context provides particular influences that are likely to impact the SR. First, the training program itself exerts an influence; in our research this was referred to as a "safety net" and a "distant presence" (Clohessy, 2008). Second, when people are in training, the role of evaluation carries particular weight as trainees/interns are aware of the possibility that they may be failed for not meeting the desired or agreed competencies of their chosen profession. Our research suggests that in effective SRs, where regular and constructive feedback is integral to supervision, evaluation is less of an issue. However, in challenging or ruptured relationships this can result in a great deal of complexity and distress, and may raise specific issues for training course staff in ethically and fairly dealing with the difficulties raised (see Chapter 8). Clearly, if a supervisee feels unsafe in their SR they are less likely to disclose difficult issues, and this has led to some interesting studies on the relationship between self-disclosure and the SR (Ladany, Hill, Corbett, & Nutt, 1996; Lemoir, 2013). Clohessy's model (2008) suggests that supervisees and supervisors bring their own histories, culture, and previous experience into supervision and that these form part of the context of the relationship. For further discussion about the contribution of supervisees and supervisors to the SR, see Chapter 3. Training contexts may also differ internationally; for example, in some countries training takes place in university-based clinics, whereas in the United Kingdom clinical training is largely embedded in National Health Service (NHS) settings.

Different working and institutional contexts also have a significant impact on the SR. For example, those working in the private sector are likely to choose their supervisors to meet their specific interests or learning styles. The contract is open to negotiation and, if the supervisor does not meet the supervisee's needs, they can end the contract and seek a more suitable arrangement. Depending on the working context, those in private practice are more likely to seek supervision for therapeutic work and the content of supervision is likely to be more case-based, that is, focused on the individual, couple, family, team, or organization with which the supervisee is working.

Those working in the public sector, such as the NHS in the United Kingdom, are often allocated internal supervisors who may also be their managers. In some professions, for example psychotherapy and counseling, the conflation of management and clinical supervision is often deemed unacceptable. Many nurses face similar dilemmas and prefer to separate out the various supervisory roles. In clinical psychology it is not uncommon to combine different aspects of supervision. For example, it is possible to be supervised by a professional line manager who offers clinical, professional, and managerial supervision. However, in recent supervision policy guidance (Division of Clinical Psychology, 2014), it is suggested that these various roles are clarified and separated. For example, line management supervision focuses on organizational objectives and monitoring of performance in relation to these objectives. The emphasis is on the quality of the service provided. This reflects the normative role of supervision and the line manager may be from a different professional group. Professional supervision focuses on professional practice standards of a particular profession, particularly in relation to ethics and codes of conduct. Discussions are likely to include continuing professional development, personal and career development plans, professional and ethical dilemmas, team working, and relationships. Professional supervision is likely to involve a more experienced practitioner from within the profession, as its primary focus is on professional development.

Clinical supervision is seen as the primary means of maintaining, updating, and developing clinical skills in assessment, formulation, and therapeutic or other interventions. The function is to ensure safe and effective practice that follows best practice in relation to theory and research. Clinical supervision may be model-specific; for example a practitioner may seek supervision to improve and develop specific therapeutic skills such as in cognitive behavioral therapy or systemic therapy. In reality, while it may be preferable to separate different aspects of supervision, it may be somewhat unrealistic in practice. Setting up three or four different SRs is time-consuming and effortful, and it is our view that several of these functions can be combined within a single SR, particularly within the same profession. There is, however, a belief that combining normative, formative, and restorative elements within the same SR is challenging. We feel, however, that this is the central core of effective supervision. Supervision is challenging and its very nature lends itself to conflict—this core dynamic provides useful opportunities for learning. The key to combining these different elements is effective contracting, not just for the work to be done but also for the SR itself. The early discussions about how the dyad will manage the dynamic between restorative, developmental, and normative, evaluative, and/or managerial functions sets the tone for effective SRs, and for inviting and reviewing feedback and progress. The key skills of contracting and feedback are discussed in detail in Chapters 6 and 7. Ethical practice and valuing difference are crucial to these discussions and are so important an area in the field of supervision that they warrant detailed consideration (see Chapter 5).

Finally, in addition to the contextual influences already mentioned (training, institutional, professional, therapeutic modality, type of work)—we should also consider the broader psychosocial, economic, and cultural contexts in which we work. These influence our practice and the SR itself. Part of the current culture within health and social care is that of evidence-based practice (Chapter 4) combined with reflective practice (Chapter 9). As authors, we are greatly influenced by our own individual personalities, identities, values and cultures, a long-term supervisory working relationship, the culture of clinical psychology in the United Kingdom, and long careers within the NHS. We share a strong belief in public service and the creative joining of reflective evidence-based and ethical practice. We believe that the SR is the most effective vehicle for the development of effective new practitioners and for maintaining the quality and skills of those who are more experienced. As such, the first part of this book will provide theory and evidence to support this proposition. The second half will focus on the how of developing and maintaining effective SRs over the professional life span. The nature of the writing will reflect these combined aims, with the first part presenting an academic and research focus and the second a more experiential, reflective, and practitioner-based focus, backed up with supervisory examples.

2

Overview of Models of Supervision and the Supervisory Relationship

The aims of this chapter are:

- to provide an overview of models and frameworks that can be used to inform supervision;
- to summarize key ideas about the supervisory relationship from these models and frameworks;
- to summarize models of the supervisory relationship.

One of the distinguishing features of applied psychology is the reciprocal interplay between theory, practice, and research. Theory provides us with a road map, a framework for formulation and making sense of experience, and guides us toward specific interventions. Our practice refines this and allows us, through reflective practice, to adapt to each client and context. Research supports the development of theory and evidence in order to improve our effectiveness. In our experience, supervisors do not always apply this fundamentally psychological framework to their supervision, relying more on personal intuition and experience. This could be because theories of supervision are not very well developed or researched. For this reason, those of us working in applied psychology tend to refer to models or frameworks of supervision, rather than theories, and these are plentiful.

Although there are many conceptual frameworks for supervision, there are few models that focus specifically on the supervisory relationship. This chapter therefore presents an overview of selected supervision models and draws out aspects that add to our understanding of the SR. We then discuss models of the SR in more detail, and review the evidence base to support them. This will include models developed from the Oxford Supervision Research Group's research on supervisees' and supervisors' experiences and perceptions of the SR. We also explore other frameworks, such as experiential learning and attachment theory, which we believe contribute to our understanding of the SR.

Models of Supervision

Supervision models are often divided into two broad categories: those developed specifically to explain the process of supervision itself, referred to as generic or supervision-specific models, and those based on psychotherapy theories

Effective Supervisory Relationships: Best Evidence and Practice, First Edition.
Helen Beinart and Sue Clohessy.
© 2017 John Wiley & Sons Ltd. Published 2017 by John Wiley & Sons Ltd.

(e.g., psychodynamic, cognitive behavior therapy). Several authors—for example, Ladany (2014), Bernard and Goodyear (2014), and Beinart (2012)—argue that there are drawbacks to using therapy models for explaining supervision. Supervision differs from therapy and is fundamentally an educational process that facilitates the learning of professional skills and roles (Holloway & Poulin, 1995; Scaife & Scaife, 2001). Many professions, not only psychology, use therapeutic models for supervision, which are not necessarily appropriate or applicable to their area of practice. Additionally, in the psychotherapy world, the use of therapy models to explain the learning process may hinder aspects of professional development and research, and may be vulnerable to boundary infringements between supervision and therapy (Ladany, 2014). Therefore, models that explain supervision itself, and models of how adults learn (e.g., Kolb, 1984), may be more useful and have become our preferred approach. However, many applied psychologists and therapists continue to use therapeutic models to guide their supervision practice. We therefore present a brief summary of these models, with a particular emphasis on their contribution to our understanding of the SR.

Supervision Models Based on Psychotherapy Models

Early accounts of supervision tended to be extrapolated from therapy models, and the majority of therapeutic schools have developed their own supervisory models. We provide a brief overview of the dominant psychotherapy models of supervision but the reader is referred to A. K. Hess, Hess, and Hess (2008) and Watkins and Milne (2014) for detailed discussion of therapy-specific models of supervision. It is worth noting that practitioners are drawn to particular therapeutic models due to how these fit with their assumptive worlds and beliefs about how people change. This is likely to affect an individual's supervision style and mode. For example, a CBT-oriented therapist or supervisor is more likely to focus on cognitions and to adopt a more structured educational stance. A humanistic orientated therapist or supervisor is likely to focus on emotions and to adopt a more experiential style. In the next section we briefly overview CBT, humanistic, psychodynamic, and systemic models of supervision.

Cognitive Behavior Therapy Models of Supervision

Beck, Rush, Shaw, and Emery (1979) set out the tenets of CBT supervision, which were subsequently developed by authors such as Liese and Beck (1997) and Padesky (1996). The underlying principles, features, and structure of supervision and therapy sessions are similar. These include a collaborative approach, use of CBT methods such as socratic questioning, and providing a clear session structure, for example, checking in, providing a bridge between sessions, agenda-setting, prioritizing, summarizing, eliciting feedback, and reviewing and setting homework. See Kennerley and Clohessy (2010) for a summary of the fundamentals of CBT supervision.

CBT supervision can be wide-ranging. Padesky (1996) developed an options grid that provides a number of foci, including mastering specific CBT skills, conceptualization, the therapeutic relationship, therapist reactions, and the supervisory process. Supervisors may also attend to their supervisee's negative thoughts and assumptions as they relate to their practice and supervision (e.g., Liese & Beck, 1997). For example, they may need to challenge supervisees' expectations of always "getting it right" in therapy.

CBT supervisors emphasize direct observation or recordings of practice and active learning methods such as role-play. Safran and Muran (2001) argue that experiential methods support experiential learning, and enable the supervisee to attend to their interpersonal responses in therapy. The emphasis on monitoring and feedback is well developed in this approach. Standardized rating scales such as the Cognitive Therapy Scale—Revised (Blackburn et al., 2001) are a useful means of assessing practice and providing feedback to the supervisee (Reiser & Milne 2012). CBT has been much researched as a therapeutic method and leads the way in evidenced-based treatments. The growth of therapy outcome research has led to manualized treatments, and the focus of supervision is often to ensure fidelity to treatment approach. Roth and Pilling (2007; 2008) have developed competency-based frameworks for the Improving Access to Psychological Therapies (IAPT) initiative in the United Kingdom. These are available online at https://www.ucl.ac.uk/pals/research/cehp/research-groups/core/competence-frameworks.

The model-specific CBT supervision competencies within this framework include: a sound knowledge of CBT theory, recognition of supervisee abilities and learning needs, the ability to structure and prioritize CBT supervision sessions, an ability to impart relevant theoretical knowledge, and communicate and model CBT skills and their application. More recently, there has been attention on assessing CBT supervision skills, including the development of the Supervisor Competence Scale (SCS, in Kennerley & Clohessy, 2010). Recent authors on CBT supervision (e.g., Newman, 2010; Reiser & Milne, 2012) have stressed more generic supervision skills and placed an emphasis on the SR for creating a safe environment for learning. Safran and Muran (2001) suggest that supervisors should monitor the quality of their SRs, and promote opportunities for experiential learning. The growth of research into CBT has not been matched by a similar amount of research into CBT supervision (Reiser & Milne, 2012). However, there is growing interest in this field, which seems particularly important for a therapy model that prides itself on its research rigor.

Psychodynamic Models of Supervision

Freud, probably the first author to write about supervision in the early 1900s, proposed an expert student model. Ekstein and Wallerstein (1972) developed this as a model of teaching and learning that emphasizes the relationships between client, therapist, and supervisor. Sarnat (2010) suggests that relationship, self-reflection, assessment, diagnosis, and intervention are central competencies for a psychodynamic therapist. She suggests that supervisors need to help supervisees become competent in three main areas—theory and technique, complex psychotherapeutic skills, and emotional and relational capacities.

The relational psychodynamic model of supervision (Frawley-O'Dea & Sarnat, 2001; Sarnat, 2012) proposes that patient–therapist and supervisee–supervisor are two reciprocally influential dyads. Exploration of the SR as it relates to the clinical relationship is seen as a central task of supervision. Both parties in the supervisory dyad introduce their transferences, anxieties, and resistances into the SR, although it is acknowledged that the supervisor has greater power and holds responsibility for establishing the frame, respecting boundaries, and attending to supervisee needs. A key aspect of this model is attending to disruptions or ruptures within the SR in order to provide the supervisee with opportunities to learn how to attend to these within the therapeutic relationship (TR). This is seen as an important way of connecting theory to lived experience, in a safe and contained SR. Integral to this model is the concept of parallel process where experiences within the TR are reflected within the SR. The supervisor's role is to address these issues and to demonstrate that emotion can be processed, leading to experiential learning. The model also suggests that supervisees can unconsciously carry unresolved organizational issues of their working and/or training contexts into the SR and that the supervisor has a role in attending to these conflicts. Unlike the earlier psychodynamic models of supervision, the relational model acknowledges the supervisor's unconscious participation and encourages collaboration and consultation to ensure that the focus stays with the supervisee's learning (Sarnat, 2012).

Humanistic Models of Supervision

There are many schools of psychotherapy that fall under the broad umbrella of humanistic modalities (e.g., person-centered, existential, and gestalt). Rogers (1957) is most well known for coining the key elements of person-centered therapy such as warmth, genuineness, empathy, congruence, and unconditional positive regard. Central to this approach of therapy and supervision is the development of the person and the conscious experiencing in the here and now of the therapy or supervisory relationship. Farber (2012; 2014) emphasizes that the relational stance of the supervisor toward the supervisee should communicate respect and attend to the development of self-awareness and the unique learning needs of the supervisee. The quality of the SR is seen as facilitative of the supervisee's learning. The supervisor is encouraged to develop an SR that is collaborative, empathic, and genuine (Farber, 2014). There is an emphasis on experiential learning, reflective practice, and emotional tone within both the SR and the TR. Emphasis is also placed on personal agency, deepening self-awareness, openness, and reflexivity. Competencies would include conceptualizing issues contextually, using phenomenological inquiry, facilitating experiential awareness, and using self as a psychotherapeutic instrument of change. In this model, the relational conditions are seen as facilitative of change, and supervisors encourage these relational conditions to promote growth and the professional development of the supervisee (Farber, 2014). Supervisor competencies include having knowledge and understanding of the supervision model; application of skills and methods; managing the SR processes; assessing and evaluating the work of the supervisee; and attending to ethical, legal, and professional issues and to difference and diversity.

Systemic Models of Supervision

There are many schools of therapy that are subsumed under systemic approaches (e.g., structural, strategic, solution-focused, narrative). The overarching framework in systemic supervision is an understanding that client, supervisee, and supervisor exist within complex systems and that there are multiple overlapping systems and perspectives within both therapy and supervision. Systemic supervision actively addresses issues of power by exploring the influences of different contexts. Rigazio-DiGilio (2014) describes the multiple contexts of systemic supervision in terms of global society, local community, supervision structure, and participants' worldviews. Systemic supervision is seen as a cultural exchange process enacted within the SR where language, thoughts, and emotions interact to form shared understandings of goals and methods in therapy and supervision. Systemic approaches are generally, but not exclusively, used within marital and family therapy. Live methods of supervision are often used, such as reflecting teams (Andersen, 1987) or family sculpts. Celano, Smith, & Kaslow (2010) describe the main features of systemic supervision as supporting the development of systemic alliances (with multiple people in the room), systemic formulation, reframing the problem, building on strengths and cohesion. A key element of this approach is holding a multidimensional, contextual, and culturally informed view of multiple perspectives within the system. One method of exploring supervisee perspective and culture is through the use of family-of-origin genograms as a way of supporting self-reflexivity and self-awareness within the therapeutic or supervisory context. Burnham (2010) has developed a useful framework to explore the multiple contextual influences within the SR (e.g., gender, race, age, ability), which will be discussed in more detail in Chapter 5. Another feature of systemic supervision is the concept of isomorphism where patterns of behavior that occur in therapeutic interactions may be mirrored in the SR (see Chapter 3).

More recently, postmodern constructivist approaches argue than meanings are co-constructed between members of a system. Narrative and solution-focused approaches fall under this umbrella. All these methods require a curiosity and capacity to focus on positive changes through co-constructing an alternative narrative. Hsu (2009) identified the following components of solution-focused supervision: a positive opening, identification of positive supervision goals, exploration of exceptions (for supervisee and client), hypothesizing, feedback, and follow-up. The supervisor often takes a consultative role and uses constructivist methods of questioning to support change (e.g., the miracle question).

In summary, we have briefly outlined the central tenets of selected psychotherapy-based models of supervision (see Table 2.1). Of note in all of the models is the importance placed on the SR. Despite the differing phenomenological approaches and assumptions of the models, all place varying degrees of emphasis on the SR as a vehicle for change and learning. A great deal of practice-based evidence supports this, and clearly there are some common factors between models. There is however, remarkably little evidence based on therapeutic modality research. We now turn to the more generic models of supervision.

Table 2.1 Summary of key features of supervision based on models of psychotherapy.

CBT	Psychodynamic	Humanistic	Systemic
• Collaborative and open SR • Structured • Mirrors structure of therapy • Can explore thoughts and assumptions of therapist as they relate to their work • Emphasis on experiential learning and feedback	• Therapy and supervision dyads seen as reciprocal (parallel process) • Exploration of SR as it relates to therapy relationship • Attending to ruptures in SR to provide learning on resolving ruptures in therapy	• Emphasis on self-awareness, personal agency, and development • Relational conditions central to change in both SR and therapy relationship • Supervisors model relational conditions	• Therapy and supervision take place in complex systems with multiple influences • Developing understanding of multiple contexts and aspects of culture on SR and therapy • Isomorphism— patterns in therapy system can be mirrored in SR

Generic or Supervision-Specific Models of Supervision

Supervision-specific models have been developed to explain the complexity of supervision (as opposed to therapy). For convenience, these are are often categorized as developmental models, (e.g., Stoltenberg, McNeill, & Delworth, 1998); social role (or task and function) models (e.g., Bernard, 1979; Carroll, 1996); and integrative models (e.g., Hawkins & Shohet, 2012; Holloway, 1995; 2014). These are discussed in more detail later in the chapter, with particular reference to the role of the SR.

Developmental Models

Developmental models of supervision became popular in the 1980s (e.g., Loganbill, Hardy, & Delworth, 1982). There are several models but all have in common an attempt to describe the professional developmental journey. Developmental models share the fundamental assumption that supervisees develop through a series of different stages and that supervisors need to adjust their supervisory style and approach to match the supervisee's level of development. (e.g., Stoltenberg, 1981). The most widely applied model—the integrated developmental model (IDM) (Stoltenberg, Bailey, Cruzan, Hart, & Ukuku, 2014)—is based on professional development in counseling and psychotherapy. This model describes four developmental levels for the supervisee and suggests how the supervisor might intervene at each level. Three "structures" are proposed (awareness of self and others, motivation, and autonomy) which represent professional development across domains of professional competence (intervention, assessment, client conceptualization, individual differences, theoretical orientation, treatment goals and plans, and professional ethics). Each phase of development is described in relation to learning needs, derived from the three central structures of awareness, motivation, and autonomy. Supervisees at level 1 are described as anxious, highly motivated, and dependent on their supervisors for advice and guidance. The primary focus is on the self while dealing with anxiety about performance and evaluation. Awareness of the other is limited. Level 2 supervisees have acquired sufficient skills and knowledge to become less internally focused and to be able to increase their focus and awareness on the client; however motivation and autonomy tend to fluctuate. Level 3 supervisees develop the ability to appropriately balance the client's perspectives and needs while maintaining self-awareness. At this level, motivation stabilizes as the supervisee begins to function relatively autonomously as a professional. In addition to addressing supervisee developmental needs, the IDM provides guidance to supervisors about how to intervene at each development level. To support level 1 supervisees, the supervisor provides structure and encourages the early development of autonomy and appropriate risk-taking. The supervisor's tasks include acting as a role model and containing anxiety. At level 2 the supervisor provides less structure and encourages more autonomy. Tasks include discussing supervisee motivation and ambivalence, modeling the professional role, and providing a more facilitative and less didactic focus. At level 3 the supervisor focuses more on personal and professional integration. The supervisor's task is to ensure consistency in performance across competence domains, identify any deficits, and work toward integration and refining a professional identity. The final level, 3i (integrated), characterizes a supervisee who has developed an integrated and individualized approach to their professional practice and has a strong awareness of their strengths and needs.

Developmental models such as the IDM, while having some intuitive appeal, lack longitudinal research to test their veracity. Additionally, development and experience per se may not necessarily lead to competence, although one is unlikely to achieve competence without some degree of experience. Rønnestad and Skovholt (2003) have conducted one of the few studies on post-qualification development and developed a model based on their qualitative work. They stress that most learning in the mental health professions occurs post-qualification. Nonetheless, there is some sound evidence for the need for direction and structure at an early phase of professional learning (Ellis & Ladany, 1997) and the development of increasing autonomy as supervisees mature (Borders, 1990). However, the need for clear structure is important across all levels of experience in dealing with a clinical crisis (Tracy, Ellickson, & Sherry, 1989) or in new SRs (Rabinowitz, Heppner, & Roehlke, 1986).

Initially, the IDM did not specify relational characteristics but more recent updates (Stoltenberg et al., 2014) emphasize the importance of the SR, and the impact of a mismatch between supervisee developmental need and supervisor intervention on the relationship in supervision.

In summary, development is endemic to supervision and there are several models that explain how individuals learn, gain experience, and develop over the professional life span. The IDM, presented here, is the most theoretically developed and has led to some supporting research (e.g., Johnston & Milne, 2012), However, the findings remain equivocal owing to a need for more longitudinal research.

Social Role Models

Social role models were developed to describe the process of supervision as distinct from therapy. They are based on the assumption that the supervisor undertakes a set of social roles that establish expectations, beliefs, and attitudes about the tasks and functions that the supervisor will perform. Typical roles for a supervisor may include teacher, consultant, assessor, and role model. Several frameworks and models of supervision incorporate the tasks and functions (role) of the supervisor, for example, Bernard (1979; 1997), Inskipp and Proctor (1993), Scaife (2009), Holloway (1995; 2014), and Hawkins and Shohet (2012). The social role models that mention the SR are summarized briefly in this section.

Inskipp and Proctor (1993)

Inskipp and Proctor (1993) developed a supervision framework describing supervisory roles that has been widely accepted in the United Kingdom (Milne & Watkins, 2014). They describe the three main roles or functions of supervision as formative, normative, and restorative. The formative function is to support a supervisee's learning and development through, for example, informing or instructing. The normative function includes the ethical, evaluative, and managerial responsibilities of the supervisor, which are likely to vary depending on the professional role, level of training and experience of the supervisee, and the nature of the supervision contract. The restorative function includes the support function of supervision and acknowledges the emotional effects of working with people who are distressed. A safe and trusting SR is important for the supervisee to be able to honestly disclose the emotional impact of the work. Inskipp and Proctor suggest that most supervision sessions will incorporate all three functions but that the focus may change according to supervisee need and level of experience.

Holloway (2014)

The systems approach to supervision (SAS) is fundamentally a relational approach to teaching the complex processes involved in supervision (Holloway, 2014). The SR is seen as the central vehicle to understanding social processes within a range of complex systems (e.g., professional context, client, supervisor, supervisee). The approach is described as collaborative problem-solving, and is characterized by a learning alliance that incorporates emotional intensity, conflict, and difference. Holloway's (1995) model builds on social role models by describing the tasks and functions of supervision but sees the supervisory relationship as central (see section on models of the SR later in this chapter) and takes into account a range of contextual factors (Figure 2.1). These contextual factors include the client, the supervisee, the supervisor, and the institution. It is proposed that seven dimensions or components of the model (relationship, client, supervisee, supervisor, institution, tasks, and function) are part of a dynamic process that interrelate and mutually influence one another (hence, the systems approach).

The SAS model addresses the complexity of the process of supervision and provides a map for analyzing a particular episode of supervision in terms of: (a) the nature of the task; (b) the function the supervisor is performing; (c) the nature

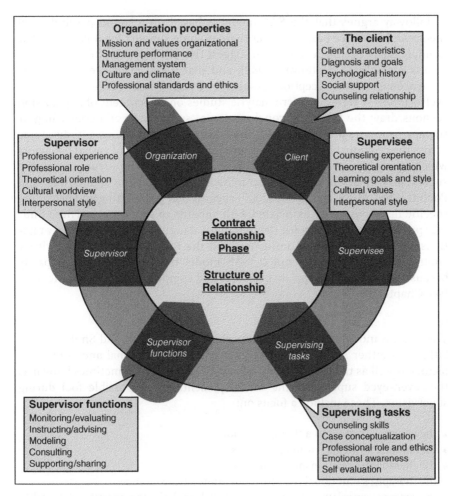

Figure 2.1 Holloway's Systems Approach to Supervision model. *Source*: Holloway 1995. Reproduced with permission of SAGE.

of the relationship; and (d) the contextual factors relevant to the process. There are numerous tasks or learning objectives of supervision identified by the model including the development of counseling skills, case conceptualization (formulation), professional role, interpersonal awareness, and self-evaluation. These could be seen as the competencies required for the development of a professional role. The five main functions or activities that the supervisor carries out during supervision are: monitoring and evaluating, instructing and advising, modeling, consulting, and supporting and/or sharing. Holloway depicts the tasks and functions of supervision as a grid. She describes the interaction of deciding what to teach (task) with how to teach it (function) as the process of supervision. The supervisee's learning needs or contextual factors (e.g., client or organizational needs) are likely to determine the supervisor role (Holloway, 2014).

Holloway argues that the SAS model is based on a sound psychological theory and evidence base, and that there is some support for this model. For example, there is some evidence to suggest that the structure of the relationship is predictable (Holloway, 1982), and that social influence factors may influence supervisor perceptions of supervisee performance (Carey, Williams, & Wells, 1988). A series of microanalytic studies on the content of supervision sessions draw the following conclusions: (a) supervision and counseling or therapy processes are distinct; (b) there are significant changes in discourse across the relationship; (c) there is a predominant pattern of verbal behaviors which resembles teacher–student interactions and the structure of the supervisory relationship has hierarchical characteristics (Holloway and Poulin, 1995). Milne and James (2000) suggest that goal-setting and providing specific instructions are associated with benefits to supervisees. These findings provide some support for the hierarchical nature of the supervisory relationship, the role of social influence, and the importance of a supervisory contract. However, the complete SAS model has not been tested, partly because of a lack of appropriate measures and complexity regarding outcomes (see Chapter 4).

Hawkins and Shohet (2012)

The process model of supervision, developed by Hawkins and Shohet (2006; 2012), is another social role model that combines relational and contextual factors as well as the tasks and functions of supervision. Sometimes known as the seven-eyed supervisor, the model presents seven possible foci during supervision. These include a focus on:

- the client or content of a therapy session;
- therapeutic strategies or interventions;
- the therapeutic relationship or process;
- the therapist's emotional reactions or counter-transference;
- the supervisory relationship and any parallels with the therapeutic relationship (parallel process);
- the impact on the supervisor or the supervisor's counter-transference; and
- the overall organizational and social context (which may include professional ethics and codes).

Hawkins and Shohet also emphasize the contracting, educational, supportive, and managerial tasks of the supervisor. This is a popular model within the United Kingdom but has had little empirical investigation. Although the SR is not conceptualized in any detail, it is one of the foci within the model and, therefore, receives some acknowledgment.

In summary, we have reviewed a range of social role models of supervision that feature the SR and have highlighted available supporting research evidence. The next section will consider other psychological models that inform our understanding of the relationship in supervision.

Other Models that Inform the Supervisory Relationship

Attachment Models

Some authors (e.g., Pistole & Watkins, 1995) suggest that the SR has the potential to incorporate elements of other important relationships, and therefore can elicit attachment responses. Supervisors can provide a secure, safe base from which supervisees can explore and develop their skills and professional identity. Pistole and Watkins (1995) suggest that an attachment bond can form between supervisor and supervisee and that elements of attachment relationships (such as safety and security) can be reflected within the SR. There is a growing body of research into attachment processes in the SR, which we shall discuss further in Chapter 3. Supervisors can be viewed as "developmental facilitators" who provide a secure base and offer encouragement, affirmation, and support, as well as facilitating supervisees' autonomy, self-efficacy, and self-worth. In summary, it has been consistently hypothesized that the concept of a safe base is an important facet of the SR in supervision. Our research, based on the measures that we have developed (see Chapter 4) finds this factor, a "safe base," to be a significant element in the conceptualization of the SR. It seems clear that a secure base is fundamental to the SR as well as core to attachment theory, but perhaps we do not yet fully understand the mechanisms underlying these relationships.

Educational and Learning Models

Supervision is an important means by which we learn for our professional and working contexts, and therefore educational and learning models provide useful frameworks for this learning. The task of the supervisor is to create a learning context that will support the needs of the supervisee, and the supervisee must engage in a way that demonstrates their "openness to learning" (Clohessy, 2008). It is beyond the scope of this chapter to comprehensively review learning models but we will cover a sample of useful models (e.g., Vygotsky and Kolb) that have influenced our understanding of the SR.

Vygotsky's zone of proximal development (ZPD) has been widely applied to supervision (e.g., James, Milne, Marie-Blackburn, & Armstrong, 2007). Vygotsky defined ZPD as "the distance between the actual developmental level as determined by independent problem solving and the level of potential development through problem solving under adult guidance or in collaboration with more capable peers" (Vygotsky, 1978, p. 86). If learning occurs within a supervisees' current developmental level, they are likely to feel unchallenged and possibly bored. If the learning challenge is beyond the ZPD of the supervisee, it is likely that they will feel out of their depth. It is therefore important that the supervisee works toward identifying and expressing appropriate learning needs and that the supervisor supports them in doing so. Several authors (e.g., Howell, 1982) discuss a progression of learning from unconscious incompetence to unconscious competence. In the initial phase of learning, supervisees are comfortable as they are unaware of what they do not know. They then become more conscious of the gaps in their knowledge and skills, which leads to a less comfortable state of conscious incompetence. There follows a phase of conscious competence where the skill becomes available to them but with conscious effort (and the support of the supervisor). The final phase is where the skill is assimilated or integrated and can be performed with unconscious competence. Clearly, a supportive and sensitive SR is required to identify appropriate goals and to negotiate a way through new learning. Models of adult learning such as Kolb's (1984; 2015) experiential learning theory recognize that adults bring into the learning environment their previous experiences and contexts. Kolb's model (Figure 2.2) proposes that learning takes place through a cycle of four stages, namely, concrete experience (experiencing), reflective observation (reflecting), abstract conceptualization (thinking), and active experimentation (doing). It is suggested that supervisees may have preferred learning styles and are most likely to enter the learning cycle through their preferred style, but will then follow the sequence through. For example, a supervisee who prefers learning by doing will engage in new learning through active experimentation and try out a method; engage in experiential learning in situ; observe and reflect on this in supervision; think about, analyze, and apply theory to make sense of the situation; and modify and test out the skill again through active experimentation.

Supervisors should be aware of supervisees' learning styles and preferences, and facilitate their learning through encouraging movement through all aspects of the learning cycle. Kolb's model has been widely applied to supervision and other professional learning contexts, and there has been research to assess preferred learning styles, leading to the development of several learning styles inventories (e.g., Honey & Mumford, 1992; Kolb, 1976). Despite some criticism of the psychometric robustness of such inventories (e.g., Cassidy, 2004), in our experience they are a useful way of initiating a conversation about learning styles and preferences, which can be helpful in establishing the SR (see Chapter 6).

So far, we have considered a wide range of models that have relevance for both supervision and the SR. The next section will explore specific models of the supervisory relationship in more detail.

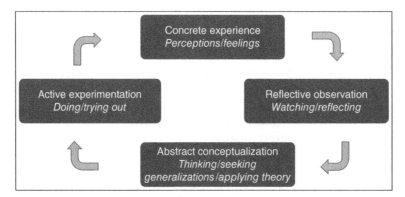

Figure 2.2 Kolb's experiential learning cycle. *Source*: Experimental Learning: Experience as the Source of Learning and Development, 2nd Ed., by Kolb, David A., ISBN 0133892409.

Models of the Supervisory Relationship

Bordin's Model of the Supervisory Working Alliance

Bordin's (1983) model of the supervisory working alliance (SWA) is based on his model of the therapeutic alliance. He describes it as a collaboration for change consisting of three aspects: (a) a mutual agreement and understanding of the goals of supervision; (b) the tasks of each of the partners in the relationship; and (c) the bond that develops between them. Bordin suggests that the clarity and mutuality of the agreement contributes to the strength of the working alliance. In addition to agreeing goals, the tasks by which each of the participants may achieve those goals also need to be negotiated. Bonds are developed through sharing a common enterprise. Indeed, Bordin suggests that time spent together; mutual liking, caring, and trusting; and the public–private dimension of the relationship influence the development of bonds. He includes the following goals of the SWA: development of specific clinical competences and an understanding of clients' and process issues; increasing awareness of self and the impact on process (therapy and supervision); overcoming personal and intellectual obstacles toward learning; deepening understanding of concept and theory; providing a stimulus to research; and maintaining professional standards.

Bordin identifies three main tasks for the supervisee. These include the preparation of oral or written reports of their work, providing opportunities for the supervisor to observe therapy, and bringing a selection of problems and issues to supervision. The supervisors' tasks include coaching, giving feedback, focusing on areas of difficulty or gaps for the supervisee, and deepening theoretical or personal understanding. The supervisory process is managed through establishing the supervisory contract and providing mutual ongoing feedback and evaluation. Bordin's model has provided an impetus for research into the alliance between supervisor and supervisee. For example, stronger SWAs have been associated with supervisee self-efficacy (Efstation, Patton, & Kardash, 1990), less role conflict and ambiguity for the supervisee (i.e., fewer competing or unclear expectations [Ladany & Friedlander, 1995]), and greater satisfaction with supervision (Ladany, Hill, Corbett, & Nutt, 1996).

In the supervision literature, the terms "supervisory working alliance" and "supervisory relationship" tend to be used interchangeably, although the SWA is a specific, theoretically driven construct based on Bordin's work on the therapeutic working alliance. As mentioned in Chapter 1, the SWA (defined as goals, tasks, and bonds) does not incorporate other important aspects of the relationship between supervisor and supervisee, including its educative, evaluative, and often involuntary nature, and the broader influences within it (such as power and culture). As such, it is a useful but partial conceptualization of some aspects of the SR.

Holloway's Model of the Supervisory Relationship in a Systems Approach to Supervision

As mentioned earlier, the SAS is the only supervision model to conceptualize the SR in any detail. Indeed, the SR is a central feature in Holloway's model: "In the systems approach to supervision, relationship is the container of a dynamic process in which the supervisor and supervisee negotiate a personal way of using a structure of power and involvement that accommodates the supervisee's progression of learning" (Holloway, 1995, pp. 41–42). Holloway identifies three essential elements of the supervisory relationship: interpersonal structure (incorporating the dimensions of power and involvement); phases of the relationship; and supervisory contracts (the establishment of a set of expectations for the tasks and functions of supervision). The interpersonal structure of the supervision relationship in this model is based on Leary's (1957) theory of interpersonal relations. This is described as power through involvement. Each individual brings to the relationship interpersonal histories that influence the level of involvement or attachment within the supervisory relationship. Although formal power rests with the supervisor, both supervisor and supervisee influence the distribution of power and the degree of attachment to one another. Holloway argues that supervisory relationships develop over time from formal to informal interpersonal relationships. In the early phase of the SR, participants rely on general sociocultural information about roles and their previous experience of hierarchical relationships. However, as more information is gathered, the relationship becomes more individualized and predictable. As the SR evolves to a more interpersonal one, there is reduced uncertainty and participants become more open and vulnerable and are more likely to self disclose. Holloway proposes three phases of development, and labels these as the beginning, mature, and terminating phases of the SR. The beginning phase involves clarifying the relationship, establishing a supervision contract, and working on specific competencies and treatment plans. During the mature phase the relationship becomes more individualized and less role-bound, which allows greater social bonding and influence. It also focuses on developing formulation skills, working on self-confidence, and exploring the personal–professional interface. The terminating phase allows increased autonomy and less need for direction from the supervisor. The supervisory contract is seen as an important means of negotiating goals and tasks, as well as of the parameters of the relationship. This clarifies both content and relational characteristics and establishes mutual expectations of the supervisory relationship.

Oxford Models of the Supervisory Relationship

The SR has been the focus of research by the Oxford Supervision Research Group, and we have developed two models that conceptualize the relationship from the perspective of the supervisor and supervisee.

Beinart's (2002; 2014) study on the SR from the perspective of the supervisee (trainee and recently qualified clinical psychologists) involved a grounded theory analysis of written answers to open-ended questions about the quality of the supervisory relationship. Nine categories were developed to describe the SR: boundaried, supportive, respectful, open, committed, sensitive to needs, collaborative, educative, and evaluative. A grounded theory was developed that proposed that a *framework* for the supervisory relationship needed to be in place for the

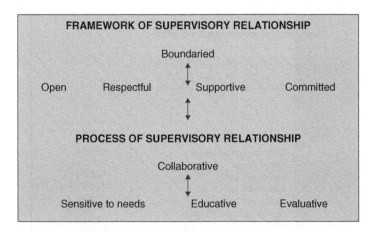

Figure 2.3 Beinart's model of the supervisory relationship (supervisee's perspective).

process or work of supervision to occur (Figure 2.3). The main aspect of the framework was the development of a boundaried relationship. This included both structural boundaries such as time, place, and frequency of supervision, and personal–professional boundaries that enabled the supervisee to feel emotionally contained within the SR. Other aspects of the framework of the relationship included the development of a mutually respectful, supportive, and open relationship where the supervisee felt the supervisor was committed to their supervision and there was regular two-way feedback between both parties. The model was influenced by Rogers's (1957) concept of necessary and sufficient conditions of therapeutic change. In supervision, certain optimal relationship conditions seem necessary for the more formal work of supervision to take place effectively.

In Beinart's study, clinical psychology supervisees described a strong preference for collaborative supervisory relationships where both parties were involved in setting the agenda and the goals of supervision. A certain amount of flexibility of approach and therapeutic model seemed to aid the collaboration. The two tasks of education and evaluation were facilitated if the supervisor was sensitive to the supervisee's needs, in terms of both their previous experience and their stage of training, as well as the personal impact of the work. Unlike previous studies (e.g., Green, 1998) the wisdom and experience of the supervisor seemed less important than opportunities to observe the supervisor's work, have stimulating discussions, and foster curiosity. The most important aspect of the educative category seemed to be collaborative work on formulation, which included theory–practice links. Again, flexibility was important to supervisees who found didactic supervision or inflexible adherence to models less helpful. Interestingly, the evaluative aspect of supervision was only an issue in poor-quality SRs where supervisees felt unsafe. Supervisees valued and appreciated feedback and challenge in strong collaborative relationships, and the formal elements of evaluation did not seem to negatively influence this.

Clohessy (2008) explored supervisors' perspectives of their SRs with trainee clinical psychologists. Using grounded theory methodology, she developed a

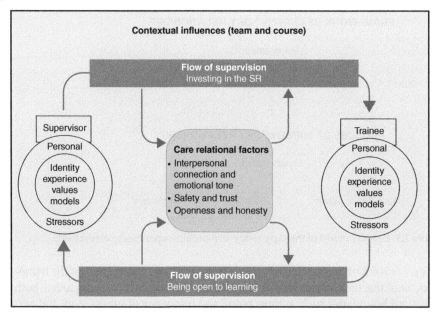

Figure 2.4 Clohessy's model of the supervisory relationship (supervisor's perspective).

model of the SR from the supervisor's perspective (Figure 2.4). She identified three categories as important in the quality of the relationship from a supervisor's perspective: contextual influences, the flow of supervision, and core relational factors. Contextual influences on the development of the relationship included the team or service within which the SR took place, the presence of the training course, and the individual factors that the supervisor and trainee bring to the relationship (such as, for example, gender, ethnicity, prior experience of supervision). The flow of supervision reflects supervisor and trainee contributions to the process of supervision. Supervisor contributions were summarized as "investing in the SR," and included ensuring a good beginning to the SR by planning ahead for the trainee, spending time together, establishing boundaries and expectations, encouraging learning, and responding to individual needs. Trainee contributions to the flow of supervision were summarized as "being open to learning" and included being enthusiastic and committed, adopting a proactive stance, and being productive. The more open to learning the trainee appeared to be, the more the supervisor invested in the relationship; this created a virtuous cycle which supported the development of positive core relational factors. The core relational factors identified in the study were the interpersonal connection between the supervisor and trainee; the emotional tone or atmosphere of the relationship; and the degree of safety, trust, openness, and honesty in the SR. The findings suggest a reciprocal relationship between these core relational factors and the flow of supervision. Although the best SRs described seemed to be characterized by positive characteristics in the three core categories identified, it seemed that SRs only needed to be "good enough" in order to work effectively.

Summary

In this chapter we have presented an overview of psychotherapy-influenced models of supervision and of supervision-specific models. We have emphasized the role of the SR within these models and discussed some models of the SR itself. We have also explored other conceptual frameworks that add to our understanding of the SR such as attachment theory and models of adult learning. We have described our own models, developed from our qualitative research. Some aspects of the models presented have received some empirical support, and by far the strongest and growing evidence base lies with the importance of the SR itself (e.g., Beinart, 2014; Ellis & Ladany, 1997). The SR is a unique relationship, which is fundamental to the effectiveness of supervision. The next chapter considers the multiple influences on the SR and the factors that contribute to more effective or less effective SRs.

Key Points

- There are numerous models and frameworks that can be used to inform supervision.
- These models and frameworks originate from the literature on psychotherapy, supervision, education, and learning.
- As supervision is fundamentally an educational process, it is important to draw on a broader range of literature than psychotherapy alone.
- Models of therapy, supervision, and education/learning vary in the emphasis they place on the supervisory relationship.
- Elements of attachment relationships may be reflected in the supervisory relationship, and a safe base has been identified as fundamental to an effective relationship in supervision.
- In models of the supervisory relationship, key features of the relationship are that it should be boundaried, safe, supportive, respectful, open, committed, sensitive to needs, collaborative, educative, and evaluative.
- Supervisors should invest in the relationship and supervisees should be open to learning through enthusiasm, curiosity, and being productive.
- Multiple contextual factors will influence the supervisory relationship in terms of the factors both supervisor and supervisee bring to the relationship (e.g., age, gender, past experience of supervision), as well as wider factors, such as the working context in which the supervisory relationship takes place.
- Power is implicit in the supervisory relationship, although both supervisor and supervisee mutually influence each other and the relationship becomes more individualized over time.

3

Influences on the Supervisory Relationship

This chapter aims:

- to summarize the multiple influences on the supervisory relationship;
- to explore these influences from the perspective of the supervisee and the supervisor, and within the contexts of the dyad and the external context.

There has been an abundance of research on the supervisory relationship. In their recent review, Inman et al. (2014) found that it was the most researched topic in the supervision literature. This is unsurprising, given the fundamental importance of the SR to effective supervision (e.g., Ellis & Ladany, 1997; Watkins 2014a). However, it is a complex relationship, comprising a dyad of supervisor and supervisee, with many contextual influences, highlighted in the models described in Chapter 2. In group supervision, these relational components and influences are even more complex. In this chapter, we will summarize the literature on the multiple influences on the SR, with special reference to what the supervisor and supervisee bring to the relationship in the context of one-to-one supervision, and other influences on the supervisory dyad.

Supervisor Contributions to the Supervisory Relationship

Supervisors contribute positively to the SR in numerous ways, in terms of the things they do in supervision, as well as through the qualities and the contextual influences they bring with them. Although there is no evidence that good therapists always make good supervisors, there is some evidence to suggest that good supervisors use therapeutic qualities in supervision. Empathy for the supervisee and client (e.g., Henderson, Cawyer, & Watkins, 1999; Nerdrum & Rønnestad, 2002), a non-judgmental stance, acceptance, and genuineness have all been highlighted as important supervisor qualities (Carifio & Hess, 1987; Hutt, Scott, & King, 1983; G. L. Nelson, 1978). A central task for supervisors involves creating a safe base in the SR (e.g., Allen, Szollos, & Williams, 1986; Clohessy, 2008; Palomo, Beinart, & Cooper, 2010) so that the supervisee is able to reflect on their

Effective Supervisory Relationships: Best Evidence and Practice, First Edition.
Helen Beinart and Sue Clohessy.
© 2017 John Wiley & Sons Ltd. Published 2017 by John Wiley & Sons Ltd.

practice and to be honest about their mistakes, their learning needs, and the personal impact of their work. In two studies that developed reliable and valid measures of the SR in UK clinical psychology, a "safe base" accounted for the largest proportion of variance in participants' scores (Palomo et al., 2010; Pearce, Beinart, Clohessy, & Cooper, 2013) reflecting the fundamental importance of safety in the SR. Supervisors can create a safe base by demonstrating the therapeutic qualities highlighted above in the context of the SR.

Another way in which supervisors can cultivate a safe, secure base in the SR is by providing appropriate boundaries for the relationship, both structural (providing uninterrupted and regular supervision) and personal or professional (supervision focused on learning needs and providing emotional containment while maintaining the boundary between supervision and therapy: Beinart, 2012). In this way, supervision becomes a protected space, with a clearly defined function. Establishing boundaries and mutual expectations has been consistently highlighted as important in the supervision literature (e.g., Holloway, 1995; Palomo et al., 2010; Scaife, 2009), and developing an effective supervision contract can make a significant contribution to this (see Chapter 6). Difficulties with boundaries and a lack of clarity in the supervision contract can be characteristic of problematic relationships (Ladany 2014; M. L. Nelson & Friedlander, 2001).

In addition, demonstrating an interest in and respect for the supervisee, collaboration, availability, and commitment to supervision have all been identified as positive supervisor contributions to the SR (Beinart, 2012; Clohessy, 2008; G. L. Nelson, 1978; Worthington, 1984). Clohessy (2008) found that a supervisor investing in the relationship was important in establishing the core relational factors of the SR (see Chapter 2). Investing in the relationship encompassed various factors such as preparing for, and spending time with, the supervisee, getting to know them, tuning into their interests and learning needs, providing constructive feedback, and encouraging reflective practice. Close monitoring and involvement at the beginning of the SR, consistency, responsiveness, sensitivity to needs and flexibility have been highlighted as ways of enabling a safe supervisory base to develop (Pistole & Watkins, 1995). Beinart (2012) found that supervisees valued supervisors who responded sensitively to their learning needs, taking into account their previous experience and stage of learning and the personal impact of the work.

Appropriate and judicious supervisor self-disclosure has been highlighted as being helpful for the supervisee, supervisor, and the SR (Knox, Edwards, Hess, & Hill, 2011). Farber (2006) suggests that the decision to disclose is a careful balancing act, and that most supervisors do so with the intention of strengthening the SR through creating an atmosphere of trust. Yourman (2003) argues that supervisor self-disclosure may ease supervisee shame and increase the supervisee's willingness to self-disclose in supervision. However, Knox et al. (2011) suggest that, although many supervisors perceive that their self-disclosure has a positive impact on their supervisee (for example, by normalizing anxiety or improving rapport), supervisees in their study viewed some supervisor disclosure as inappropriate and suggested that it could lead to a loss of credibility. Arguably, supervision relies on the supervisor's ability to share relevant information with the supervisee, that is, pertinent material that will enhance supervisee learning. However, the broader literature suggests that it can be common for supervisors not to share highly relevant feedback with the supervisee, for example, a negative reaction to supervisee skills or performance. Often this may be for reasons such as an assumption that the supervisee will discover the issue for themselves, or that such feedback is somehow irrelevant to the goals of supervision or perhaps reflects the supervisor's own issues. Some supervisors may be concerned about turning supervision into a therapy session, or that their disclosure may give rise to a negative reaction (Ladany & Melincoff, 1999). However, there is a general consensus in the literature that certain issues, such as sexual attraction to the supervisee, should not be disclosed (Ladany, Constantine, Miller, Erickson, & Muse-Burke, 2000; Skjerve et al., 2009). More research into supervisor (non-)disclosure is needed, as well as into the impact that supervisor disclosure has on the supervisee and the SR.

Supervisors can also contribute to problems in the relationship. Imbalanced, developmentally inappropriate supervision; an inability to manage boundaries or feedback or to clarify expectations effectively; and intolerance of differences have all been identified as problematic supervisor behaviors (Magnuson, Wilcoxon, & Norem, 2000; Ramos-Sánchez et al., 2002). Misuse of power, resulting in boundary infringements or poor ethical practice (see Chapter 5) have also been highlighted as particularly relevant in contributing to problems in the SR (Falender & Shafranske, 2004). Such difficulties can compromise the ability of the supervisor to monitor the treatment of the client, particularly if the supervisee is unable to be open about their learning needs, uncertainties, or mistakes; their emotional responses to their clients; or their feelings about the supervision itself. The literature has described as ineffective or harmful, supervisors who were uninterested in supervision or the supervisee, were unavailable (McCarthy, Kulakowski, & Kenfield, 1994); were too authoritarian (Cherniss & Egnatios, 1977); were perceived as critical and unsupportive (Hutt, Scott, & King, 1983); provided the supervisee with too little feedback; were indirect or avoidant (Wulf & Nelson, 2001), inflexible, intolerant, or defensive (Watkins, 1997).

Contextual factors are important when considering influences on the SR. Each member of the dyad will bring unique aspects of difference and diversity that influence their identities and the SR. The most widely studied aspect of diversity explored in the literature is the impact of race and ethnicity on the SR. However, the results from racial matching in supervisory dyads are inconclusive (Inman et al., 2014). Creating a climate whereby issues of difference and diversity can be explored is an important supervisor responsibility, although research suggests that conversations about cultural issues occur relatively infrequently in supervision, and supervisors rarely initiate them (Inman et al., 2014). Supervisors' awareness of their own cultural identity and assumptions, and of how these may influence supervision, are particularly important both in terms of reducing the risk of micro-aggressions when working with culturally different supervisees, and in creating a climate where race and culture can be explored safely in supervision (Inman et al., 2014). Initiating supportive discussions about culture have been shown to be related to supervisee self-efficacy and to greater satisfaction with supervision (e.g., Ng & Smith, 2012). Supervisors with racial consciousness higher than or on a par with that of their supervisees were better at creating relationships in which multicultural competence could develop, and had stronger working alliances.

Similarly, the impact of the supervisor's gender as a contextual influence on the SR has attracted some research and some interesting findings. The gender of the supervisee (and of the client) elicits particular expectations that can influence supervision (Doughty & Leddick, 2007). Similarly, there may be expectations about the supervisor based on gender. Female supervisors are expected to be more nurturing while male supervisors are often viewed as "experts" and to focus more on the appropriateness of the supervisee's actions (Doughty & Leddick, 2007). Much of the literature in this area suggests that men and women perceive each other within traditional gender role contexts, which in turn influences the SR. These influences may be positive or negative. For example, research suggests that both male and female supervisors are less likely to reinforce female supervisees' attempts to take on a more powerful role (M. L. Nelson & Holloway, 1990), are more likely to tell their female supervisees what to do (Granello, Beamish, & Davies, 1997), and ask male supervisees for their opinions twice as often as female supervisees. Interestingly, male supervisors perceived that they had formed good relationships with both male and female supervisees (Worthington & Stern, 1985). Warner (1998) describes the gendered constructs of expressiveness and instrumentality in communication styles in supervision. Expressiveness is traditionally associated with feminine characteristics of empathy and intimacy in relationships, whereas instrumentality has been associated with traditional masculine characteristics such as goal direction, independence, and self-confidence. Warner found that supervisor expressiveness was positively correlated with working alliance, supervisor impact, and supervisee disclosure, whereas supervisor instrumentality seemed to be helpful in developing supervisee self-efficacy. Given that gender is an important (and rarely addressed) contextual influence on the SR, supervisors need to remain mindful and aware of these influences and to support an environment where gender issues can be explored and discussed (Doughty & Leddick, 2007; Gatmon et al., 2001), including a willingness to consider their own biases, expectations, style of communication, as well as the influence on power within the relationship.

Ethnicity and gender are the cultural influences on the SR that have received most attention in the supervision literature. It's important to note that there are other aspects of difference that may need consideration (such as spirituality, sexual orientation, disability), which have received less attention in the research literature. For example, supervisor homophobic attitudes have been associated with supervisees' reduced satisfaction with supervision, regardless of the sexual orientation of the supervisee (Harbin, Leach, & Eells, 2008). It is important that supervisors are able to model sensitive and affirmative practice and are open and comfortable in addressing issues of sexual orientation. It is also important that they support LGBTQ supervisees in managing issues of homophobia in their work settings (Burkard, Knox, Hess, & Schultz, 2009; Messinger, 2007; Satterly & Dyson, 2008). Again, the task for the supervisor is to create a SR in which aspects of difference and their influence on the SR and on the supervisee's work can be explored.

Table 3.1 Summary of supervisor contributions to effective supervisory relationships.

- Creation of a safe space in the SR through establishing boundaries and mutual expectations
- Use of therapeutic qualities such as empathy, respect, genuineness, and acceptance
- Interest and investment in the SR; being available to the supervisee
- Collaborative attitude
- Flexibility and responsiveness to needs
- Appropriate self-disclosure
- Provision of feedback to the supervisee
- Awareness of difference and diversity, and ability to initiate supportive discussions.

Supervisors bring other factors to the relationship that may influence supervision (Table 3.1). These include personal and/or professional beliefs, ethical practice, working contexts, and prior experience of supervision. Clohessy (2008) found that SRs tended to work better for supervisors who felt more experienced and confident in the supervisory role. Learning and reflecting on their own experience as a supervisee was also valuable for some supervisors in developing their own supervisory style. Additionally, personal stressors such as poor health or coping with difficult life events can also impact on and distract attention from the SR for both parties.

Supervisee Contributions to the Supervisory Relationship

There has been some interesting research on supervisee contribution to the SR. Vespia, Heckman-Stone, and Delworth (2002) identified the characteristics of counseling psychology supervisees who make good use of supervision. These included acceptance of feedback, a willingness to grow, listening to the supervisor, able to tolerate uncertainty, and to critique their own work. Norem, Magnuson, Wilcoxon, and Arbel (2006) suggested that the supervisees who made best use of supervision were mature, autonomous, knowledgeable, open to experience, and self-aware. Clohessy's (2008) study highlighted that supervisors identify supervisees' openness to learning as an important contribution to the SR. This included behaviors such as demonstrating enthusiasm, commitment, a proactive stance (being active participants in supervision rather than passive recipients), and working hard (see Table 3.2).

Kauderer and Herron (1990) identified that supervisors value supervisees who were assertive, less dependent, and clear about the differences between supervision and therapy. Those who were able to form good relationships in the work context, were flexible and sensitive to ethical issues, and were reflective of their emotional responses to their practice were also seen as the "best" supervisees. Vespia et al. (2002) suggest that supervisors value supervisees who listen to and act on supervisors' instructions, particularly when there are concerns for client welfare. Falender and Shafranske (2012) confirm that, for supervisees to get the most out of supervision, they need to take responsibility for the preparation of material for supervision, to be open to discussions and learning, to report honestly on their actions, and to follow through supervisory guidance.

Table 3.2 Summary of supervisee contributions to effective supervisory relationships.

- Openness to learning: receptiveness to feedback and willingness to be open about their work
- Proactive stance: hard-working, committed, enthusiastic, assertive, mature, and appropriate autonomy
- Ethical awareness
- Self-awareness and self-reflectivity
- Ability to critique own work
- Ability to form good relationships in working contexts.

Supervisees also bring a multitude of contextual influences to the SR. We have already discussed the impact of supervisor gender on the relationship but, of course, the supervisee's gender influences the SR too. As mentioned earlier, female supervisees are more likely to be told what to do and less likely to be encouraged to adopt a powerful role by supervisors of either gender. Male supervisees are more likely to *believe* that they have formed closer SRs with their supervisors (Worthington & Stern, 1985) and more likely to focus on issues to do with the client (rather than on their own learning and development, or their feelings about their work (Sells, 1993). Female supervisees have been found to place more emphasis on relationship variables in supervision, whereas male supervisees are more task-focused in supervision. The research evidence on same- versus mixed-gender pairings in supervision is mixed (Doughty & Leddick, 2007). Once again, it seems that it is important to create a relationship whereby contextual influences such as gender can be acknowledged and explored.

A supervisee's willingness to be open with their supervisor about their work is a prerequisite for effective supervision and an important aspect of productive learning (Alonso & Rutan, 1988). Yet it is not always easy for supervisees to self-disclose in this way. Mehr, Ladany, and Caskie (2010) reported that 84% of supervisees in their study said that they had not disclosed information in a recent supervision session

Many supervisees find it difficult to be open in supervision, and there has been some research into why this is the case. Unsuprisingly, a poor supervisory alliance is a common reason (S. A. Hess et al., 2008; Inman et al., 2011; Ladany et al., 1996). Perceived unimportance of the issue (Inman et al., 2011; Ladany et al., 1996), fear of negative evaluation, and feelings of shame have also been highlighted as reasons supervisees choose not to disclose in supervision (S. A. Hess et al., 2008; Inman et al., 2011; Reichelt et al., 2009; Yourman, 2003). Anxiety may be another reason for supervisee non-disclosure, whether anxiety about upsetting the supervisor or of damaging the SR (Inman et al., 2011; Reichelt et al., 2009) or anxiety about their own performance and skills (S. A. Hess et al., 2008; Mehr et al., 2010). Power in the SR may also influence the degree of self-disclosure by supervisees (S. A. Hess et al., 2008) who may prefer to disclose in another less hierarchical relationship, for example to a peer, another professional, or a friend (Inman et al., 2011; Ladany et al., 1996).

The *content* of supervisee self-disclosure has also been the subject of research interest. The most common issues supervisees do not share relate to negative reactions to the supervisor or to the supervision experience, personal issues, and clinical mistakes. Feeling unable to raise concerns about supervision or about the supervisor is perhaps unsurprising, given the hierarchical nature of the SR. Non-disclosure of personal issues that may impact on the supervisee's work is more concerning. However, not disclosing clinical mistakes is particularly worrying if we consider the quality control function of supervision and that good client outcomes are an important goal. Other non-disclosures may be related to evaluation concerns, general observations about clients, countertransference, negative reactions or sexual attraction to clients, supervisor appearance, and attraction to the supervisor (Ladany et al., 1996; Lemoir, 2013; Mehr et al., 2010).

Dyadic Influences

So far, we have looked at research into the multiple factors that both supervisor and supervisee contribute to the SR. This section focuses on other influences on the supervisory dyad—namely, attachment processes, client-related influences and factors (such as parallel process or isomorphism), power, and external contextual factors such as the service or organizational context in which the SR takes place.

Attachment Processes in the Supervisory Relationship

Attachment models (see Chapter 2) have been widely applied to a range of different relational contexts, including the SR. Attachment processes have become the focus of research interest in the SR since the mid-1990s. Neswald-McCalip (2001, p. 22) suggests that the attachment relationship in supervision "provides the supervisee with sufficient safety so that he or she feels confident addressing the supervisor in times of crisis." Providing a secure supervisory base and a safe haven can therefore be seen as an important way in which the supervisor can enhance learning (e.g., Bennett & Saks, 2006; Pistole & Watkins, 1995; Watkins, 1995). Supervisees may show attachment styles in supervision similar to their attachment patterns in other close relationships (Foster, Lichtenberg, & Peyton, 2007). Researchers have suggested that the challenges of the supervision experience may activate the attachment system so that the supervisee seeks closeness and safety from the supervisor (Bennett, 2008). Bennett and Deal (2009) found that secure attachment style in supervision was related to supervisee self-reflection, meta-cognitive processing, empathy, and the ability to recognize the subjectivity of perceptions. Bennett and Vitale Saks (2006) suggest that supervisees with secure attachment styles may develop working models of others as reliable and consistent, and so be more likely to ask for help, accept feedback, and explore new learning opportunities. However, there is some suggestion in the literature that general attachment style is less important than relationship-specific attachment style (Bennett, 2008). So, for example, a supervisee may have a generally secure attachment style but become distant with a supervisor whom they perceive to be unsupportive. Foster et al. (2007) found that supervisees with insecure attachments to their supervisor perceived themselves as being at lower levels of professional development, compared with those who were securely attached. Avoidant or dismissing attachment styles in supervisees can be particularly problematic in supervision, particularly compulsive self-reliance, which involves interpersonal strategies such as distancing, extreme autonomy, distrust, and fear of depending on others (e.g., Bennett, Mohr, BrintzenhofeSzoc, & Saks, 2008). The literature suggests that supervisees with insecure attachment patterns may use affect regulation strategies in the face of stressful situations in their work and/or supervision. These are characterized by distancing (if avoidant, for example, minimizing distress or the importance of an event) or dependency (if anxiously attached, for example, exaggerating distress, seeking closeness and approval). As such, it is important that supervisors are aware of this and respond accordingly (e.g., Pistole & Fitch, 2008; Watkins & Riggs 2012). The suggestion that supervisee insecure attachment style is associated with a negative outcome in supervision has received partial support in the literature (Bennett et al., 2008; Deal, Bennett, Mohr, & Hwang, 2011; Foster et al., 2007; Renfro-Michael & Sheperis, 2009), but further research is needed (Watkins & Riggs, 2012). Some studies have also explored the role of early experience on attachment dynamics in the SR, and there is some suggestion that parental indifference may lead to maladaptive attachment behaviors that have a negative impact on supervision (Dickson, Moberly, Marshall, & Reilly, 2011; Riggs & Bretz, 2006).

Given the dyadic nature of the SR, *supervisor* attachment processes have also been explored. V. E. White and Queener (2003) found that it was the supervisors' (rather than the supervisees') ability to make adult attachments that was predictive of both the supervisors' and supervisees' perceptions of the working alliance. In other words, a significant proportion of the supervisory working alliance was predicted by the supervisors' ability to form close relationships. In another study, Riggs and Bretz (2006) explored the impact of attachment processes on the SR by surveying 86 experienced clinical and counseling psychology trainees, and found that the supervisees' perception of their supervisors' attachment style had the most direct impact on the supervisory alliance. Their study, which compared dyads that consisted of insecure supervisors and secure or insecure supervisees and dyads that consisted of secure supervisors with secure or insecure supervisees, found that the former were characterized by problematic supervisory alliances. Dickson et al. (2011) reported similar findings in their study, with supervisees who reported lower ratings of their working alliances when they perceived their supervisor to be insecurely attached.

In a recent examination of the small but influential literature on attachment processes in supervision, Watkins and Riggs (2012) suggest that the SR is best viewed as involving an affective component that can trigger attachment dynamics, rather than as a true attachment relationship. These relationships may be too brief in duration, and have a different function and purpose to other relationships in which attachment has been seen as relevant (such as romantic relationships). Some SRs may, however, be deemed as more akin to full attachment relationships, particularly if they are of longer duration and occur earlier in the supervisee's professional development, when anxiety and dependency are high. However, Watkins and Riggs suggest that attachment dynamics in the SR are best conceptualized in the context of a leader–follower attachment relationship, which better reflects the role and function of the SR. The work or learning context is seen as very different to early family attachments, in that it is short-term and mutually influenced by context and the early experiences of both parties. In the leader–follower model, supervisors are seen as "developmental facilitators" who empower their supervisees by offering affirmation, encouragement, and support (Mayseless, 2010). They also stimulate and motivate their supervisees to work toward greater autonomy and a sense of self-worth and self-efficacy. Mayseless (2010) found that securely attached leaders were more able to promote these characteristics in their followers by offering a consistent and responsive secure base.

In summary, the literature on attachment processes and the SR provides an interesting and useful perspective on dynamics in the relationship. The research in this area is small and has some limitations (e.g., reliance on self-report measures and supervisees' assessment of their supervisors' attachment style). However, further research is warranted; Watkins and Riggs (2012) provide some helpful suggestions for future research, conceptualizing attachment in the context of leader–follower relationships.

Parallel Process and Isomorphism

Parallel process is a popular concept in the supervision literature, and is particularly relevant in some psychodynamic and process-informed models (e.g., Frawley-O'Dea, 2003; Hawkins and Shohet, 2012; see Chapter 2). It refers to the mirroring of aspects of the therapeutic relationship in the SR and vice versa. Theoretically, parallel process is an intrapsychic phenomenon that occurs unconsciously and originates in a relationship in one setting that is reflected in a relationship in another setting. For example, a therapist working with a client experiencing feelings of being stuck and hopeless may mirror this in the supervisory relationship with their supervisor. Despite its popularity as a concept in understanding processes in supervision, there is little in the way of research in this field. Tracey, Bludworth, and Glidden-Tracey (2012) found evidence of parallel process in the interaction patterns of supervision triads (including supervisor, supervisee, and client), and that this was a bi-directional process—aspects of the SR were also mirrored in the therapeutic relationship (TR). However, Jacobsen (2007) suggests that the pattern of interaction and parallels between the SR and the TR is more complicated than a simple bi-directional relationship.

Although it is similar to parallel process, isomorphism is a relational concept used in systemic understanding as opposed to an intra-psychic construct used in psychodynamic explanations. M. B. White and Russell (1997) recognize that patterns that emerge between supervision and practice are bi-directional and can emerge from practice to supervision or from supervision to practice. Koltz, Odegard, Feit, Provost, and Smith (2012) describe isomorphism as a repetitive relational pattern that occurs in supervision, and that the focus on a recurrent relational pattern separates isomorphism from parallel process.

Watkins (2010) cautions against assuming that all similarities between the SR and TR are parallel processes, and suggests that sometimes processes can simply occur in parallel that do not benefit from a full parallel process explanation. We agree that it may at times be "convenient" to explain SR difficulties as parallel process and thus avoid real issues of difference within the dyad. See Chapter 8 for further discussion of managing difficult issues in the SR.

Although both concepts are often used interchangeably in the literature, it is important for supervisors to be aware of the different interventions that may be needed and not to assume that all relational similarities are parallel processes. The research is currently limited but use of these concepts is widespread and is supported by practice experience.

External Contextual Factors

In addition to supervisor and supervisee factors, there are wider contextual factors that may influence the SR. However, there is little empirical research on wider contextual influences on the SR, even though these are highlighted in some supervision models (e.g., Hawkins & Shohet, 2012; Holloway 1995). In research from the Oxford Supervision Research Group, external contextual factors, such as the service within which the SR takes place and (if the supervisee is in training) the training course, were highlighted as having an influence on the SR. In a qualitative study on the SR, the working context was highlighted as important to experienced supervisors. The relationships between the supervisee and other professionals in the service could impede or facilitate the relationship between the supervisor and supervisee. Some supervisors described making efforts to establish their own relationships with their colleagues, so if a supervisee invested in these team relationships too it was valued or appreciated and, in turn, it facilitated the SR. Conversely, if supervisees were not respectful of these relationships and did not make efforts to get to know the team, it could impede the SR. The team response to the supervisee was also highlighted as positively influencing the SR in this study, with team colleagues investing in the relationship with the supervisee by contributing to their learning, and valuing them for their contribution. Some supervisors suggested that if the service context was unwelcoming, or was an unsupportive context for supervisee learning, it could negatively influence the SR between supervisor and supervisee. In this study, the SRs were training relationships, and for most supervisors the training course was another relevant contextual influence. Supervisors valued the course as a background rather than a foreground influence, and valued the knowledge of the "distant presence" of the training program should there be problems in the SR (Clohessy, 2008).

There are other contextual factors that could influence the SR, such as the broader sociopolitical environment, but to our knowledge there has been no research exploring these as yet. However, considering the impact of a range of contextual factors may help in formulating difficulties in the SR. This will be discussed in Chapter 8.

Conclusions

In this chapter we have considered the literature on the multiple influences on the supervisory dyad. We have reviewed the contributions that both supervisor and supervisee make to the SR, which we hope will provide a guide to helpful (and less helpful) behaviors in supervision. We have also presented literature on other potential influences on the dyad, including contextual factors, as well as psychological processes such as attachment, parallel process, and isomorphism. It is important to be mindful of these influences, particularly in ensuring that the SR works well and in making sense of any difficulties that may arise. In the next chapter, we consider how to assess the quality of the SR and the issues implicit in assessing a range of outcomes associated with supervision.

Key Points

- The supervisory relationship is a complex relationship that is influenced by multiple factors including the supervisor, the supervisee, the dyad, and the external context.
- Supervisors contribute to effective supervisory relationships by investing in the relationship through flexibility and responsiveness and by establishing boundaries and being sensitive to difference and diversity.
- Supervisees contribute to effective supervisory relationships by being open to learning, taking a proactive stance, reflecting on their practice, and being sensitive to ethical issues in their work.
- Other influences on the relationship include dyadic contributions (e.g., parallel process, isomorphism, attachment processes) and external contextual factors such as the training course or work environment.

4

Outcomes and Measurement

The aims of this chapter are:

- to summarize a range of supervision competencies and supervision outcomes;
- to summarize key measures of the supervisory relationship;
- to describe how regular client outcome measures can provide a structure and focus of supervision.

How do we assess the effectiveness of supervision and decide on appropriate outcomes? This has been a challenge for researchers in the field over many years. We argue throughout this book that research in supervision is limited and, with some exceptions, of generally poor quality. There are several reasons for this, and it is beyond the scope of this chapter to provide a full analysis, but the reader is referred to Ellis, D'Iuso, and Ladany (2008), Falender (2014a), and Olds and Hawkins (2014) for detailed discussions of research and measurement in supervision. Increased interest in this subject is reflected by a recent issue of *Training and Education in Professional Psychology* (Falender, 2014b), which is entirely devoted to supervision outcomes. This is encouraging but many of the authors conclude that we are still a long way off understanding what is effective in clinical supervision and that this is impeding our study of outcomes (Falender, 2014a). Consequently, there has been a great deal of recent work on agreeing and developing competency standards and operationalizing knowledge, skills and attitudes to deliver effective supervision.

Olds and Hawkins (2014) conducted an international thematic analysis and identified nine themes representing consensus on specific competencies necessary for effective supervision, as shown in Table 4.1. Additionally, the American Psychological Association (APA) has recently published guidance for supervision that covers seven similar competencies, which are outlined in Table 4.2.

This chapter focuses on the diverse range of supervisory outcomes and reviews measures of the supervisory relationship. We will also provide a brief summary of the evidence for the various outcomes ranging from supervisee satisfaction to client outcome. We do know that supervisees value supervision, and it is often rated as the most valuable aspect of training (e.g., Rakovshik & McManus, 2013; Scott, Pachana, & Sofronoff, 2011). However, to justify the time and effort invested in supervision we need to be able to show that it makes a difference to

Effective Supervisory Relationships: Best Evidence and Practice, First Edition.
Helen Beinart and Sue Clohessy.
© 2017 John Wiley & Sons Ltd. Published 2017 by John Wiley & Sons Ltd.

Table 4.1 Thematic analysis of supervisor competency frameworks.

Ethical and professional practice
Knowledge of the profession
Diversity
Reflective practice
Supervisory alliance
Structuring supervision
Supervision research and theory
Learning and evaluation

Source: Old 2014. Reproduced with permission of APA.

Table 4.2 Guidelines for Clinical Supervision in Health Service Psychology.

Domain A: Supervisor competence
Domain B: Diversity
Domain C: Supervisory relationship
Domain D: Professionalism
Domain E: Assessment/evaluation/feedback
Domain F: Problems of professional competence
Domain G: Ethical, legal, and regulatory considerations

Source: American Psychological Association, 2014. Reproduced with permission of APA.

supervisee learning and that it benefits the supervisee's clients. In fact, it is quite surprising that while, in the majority of helping professions supervision is fundamental to training and continuing professional development, we do not have an established research base to clearly articulate how and why it is effective. However, what we do know is that the SR is pivotal to the process of change and supervision outcomes (Watkins, 2014a). Regardless of the type of supervision provided, the client group, or the service context, the SR is recognized as essential in making the work of supervision effective. As is evident in the competency frameworks mentioned, the development and maintenance of the SR is seen as a core competence in supervision.

What Do We Mean by Supervision Outcomes?

For many years, client change has been held up as the gold standard of supervision outcome (e.g., Ellis & Ladany, 1997). Of course, this is incontestable; all those in the helping professions would agree that improving the quality of life for those that access their services is the fundamental goal of supervision. Supervisors should aim to support, monitor, maintain, and improve the quality of the supervisees' performance, the aim of which is to improve the service to the client and to enhance client outcome. However, there are many variables that influence what happens between supervision and client outcome. These include the competence of the supervisor, the quality and nature of the SR, supervisee training and learning, changes to supervisee awareness, behavior and skills, the supervisees' well-being and satisfaction, the relationship between supervisee and their client, the choice and quality of the intervention, and countless cultural and contextual factors. We and other authors (e.g., Bernard & Goodyear, 2014; Watkins, 2014a) argue that the SR mediates all of the above factors. Much of the literature (e.g., Ladany & Inman, 2008; Wheeler & Richards, 2007) has raised the complexity of research in this area. In order to enhance our understanding we need robust measures of the SR and to be clear about which supervision outcomes we are measuring. In the next section, we discuss the evidence for a range of supervision outcomes, after which we shall focus on specific measures of the SR. (The reader is directed to Watkins and Milne [2014, part 4] for a discussion of general supervision measures.)

Impact on the Supervisee

This section summarizes the evidence base for the SR in relation to a range of potential outcomes. It is clear from the evidence that supervision has an effect on supervisees. It is also important to note that this effect is not always beneficial and that supervisees have both positive and negative experiences that can last for many years after a SR has ended (Ellis et al., 2014; Ladany, 2014).

Satisfaction with Supervision

There is reasonably strong evidence that a positive SR is predictive of supervisee satisfaction with supervision (Ladany, Ellis, & Friedlander, 1999). It has been suggested that satisfaction with supervision is likely to reflect a supervisory experience where the SR has met supervisee expectations. Similarly, low supervisee satisfaction can be seen as a proxy measure of a poor SR (O'Donovan & Kavanagh, 2014). Low satisfaction has been found to influence a range of factors such as supervisee non-disclosure (Ladany et al., 1996), supervisee sense of self-efficacy (Cashwell & Dooley, 2001), and confidence (Bambling, 2000). Although much research has used satisfaction as an outcome measure, there has been long-standing concern about relying exclusively on this as an indicator of successful supervision because supervisees may experience some dissatisfaction with their most effective SRs. An effective SR should challenge and stretch supervisee development, which may not always feel comfortable and may result in lower ratings of satisfaction. There is a danger that satisfaction may not reflect other aspects of supervision outcome such as supervisee skill development and behavior change. In other words, satisfaction with supervision, although important, may not be an adequate or sufficient measure of supervision effectiveness.

Supervisee Knowledge, Learning, and Development

Research suggests that supervision has a positive impact on supervisees including greater self-awareness. For example, in a qualitative study supervisees reported that they were more aware of their motivation as a result of supervision (Borders, 1990). Raichelson, Herron, Primavera, and Ramirez's (1997) study of parallel process suggested that supervisees felt that supervision contributed to a deeper awareness of their subjective emotional responses to clients.

Borders (1990) also reported that supervision had a number of other positive impacts on supervisees, including enhanced treatment knowledge, skill acquisition, and more consistent application of skills. Additionally, facilitative conditions in the SR, such as empathy and warmth, were found to be positively related to supervisee skill development (Schacht, Howe, & Berman, 1989). More recent research (Bambling & King, 2014) found that positive SRs reflected supervisors' interpersonal skills and both technical and interpersonal skill development in the supervisee. Mannix et al. (2006), in a study of cognitive behavioral therapy (CBT) supervision, also reported increased competence, self-awareness, and self-efficacy in supervisees. Worthen and McNeill (1996) additionally found that enhanced formulation skills were supported by a positive SR.

Patton and Kivlighan (1997) found that the quality of the SR affected the quality of the supervisee–client alliance and enhanced knowledge and understanding of therapeutic relationships. In their study, week-to-week fluctuations in the SR accounted for a substantial portion of week-to-week fluctuations in supervisees following the agreed treatment model (brief psychodynamic therapy).

Self-efficacy

Bandura (1986) defined self-efficacy as the degree to which individuals consider themselves capable of performing a particular activity. It has been argued that supervisees' beliefs in their own efficacy improve outcomes, and a few studies have explored this notion. Cashwell and Dooley (2001) and Whittaker (2004) found that counselors who received supervision reported higher rates of self-efficacy. Ladany and Lehrman-Waterman (1999) also found that effective evaluation processes were related to higher ratings of the SR and self-efficacy. Efstation et al. (1990) found a strong correlation between self-efficacy, rapport, and task focus within the SR and aspects of supervisor style. More recently, Crockett and Hays (2015) describe a relationship between supervisor multicultural competence, the SR, and supervisee experience of self-efficacy and satisfaction with supervision. However, the findings in this area are somewhat equivocal, with suggestions that supervision impacts self-report of self-efficacy for novice supervisees but may be less significant for more experienced practitioners.

Well-being

There is some significant research showing the impact of supervision on staff well-being, job satisfaction (Kavanagh et al., 2003), and staff retention. A positive or more highly rated SR has been found to relate to increased supervisee well-being, greater job satisfaction, decreased burnout, and enhanced supervisee coping resources. Conversely, where SRs have been rated as poor by supervisees, findings suggest that this relates to reduced well-being and job satisfaction and higher supervisee anxiety, stress, burnout, role conflict, and ambiguity (Watkins 2014a; 2014b). E. White and Winstanley (2010) also found that in health service contexts supervision reduced burnout and increased staff retention.

Many who work in the helping professions find their work demanding and stressful (Hannigan, Edwards, & Burnard, 2004). Often this is exacerbated by increased demand and complexity, organizational change, and lack of support. Interestingly, there are a few studies that suggest that high-quality supervision can act as a protective factor and buffer for work-related stress, and increase staff resilience. Bakker, Demerouti, and Euwema (2005) found that a positive SR, social support, a sense of autonomy, and regular feedback decreased the risk of staff burnout, regardless of the stress of the job. Similarly, Cushway and Tyler (1994) found that psychologists rated support from colleagues as the most likely factor to alleviate stress. Howard (2008) argues that the application of positive psychology to clinical supervision is a promising approach to increase job satisfaction, performance, and well-being for staff who work in inherently challenging environments. Although there is not a great deal of evidence to support the argument that supervision enhances staff resilience, it is certainly an area that merits further investigation.

Impact on Clients

One of the major challenges facing researchers in this field is in tracking the impact of supervision and the SR on client outcome. Ellis and Ladany (1997) conducted the first review of the area (nine studies) and concluded that, owing to methodological constraints, "few justifiable conclusions" could be drawn. Freitas (2002) presented an expanded review (14 studies) and developed some pointers for future research. Other reviews, such as Wheeler and Richards (2007) and Inman and Ladany (2008), have also drawn attention to the complexity of researching client outcomes. Watkins (2011a) undertook a further review, building on previous work, and identified 18 papers covering the period 1981–2011. However, on close analysis, he concluded that the majority of papers did not actually assess client outcome but, rather, covered areas such as parallel process, therapist behavior, psychotherapy skills training, and ability to form positive therapeutic relationships. Other studies reflected counselors' opinion of client change but did not measure the impact of supervision or the SR on therapeutic change. Watkins (2011a) concluded that only three studies—Bambling et al. (2006); Bradshaw, Butterworth, and Mairs (2007), and E. White and Winstanley (2010)—actually investigated the impact of supervision on client outcome. Although they are not without methodological challenges, these studies will be described in more detail. We shall also explore an emerging area of client session-by-session feedback and how it relates to the SR.

Bambling et al. (2006) conducted the most robust study to date comparing supervised and unsupervised practice and examining a range of client outcome variables such as treatment completion and reduction of depressive symptoms in a group of 127 clients with a diagnosis of major depression. Both supervisors and supervisees were experienced psychologists or social workers, and eight sessions of supervision were provided using both supervision manuals and treatment manuals for problem-solving therapy. Supervisees were randomly assigned to one of three supervision conditions: alliance skill focus (following a

CBT approach), alliance process focus (following a psychodynamic framework), and no supervision. There were no significant differences between the two supervision groups, but there were significant differences between supervised and unsupervised practice on a range of client outcome variables. These included higher ratings of the therapeutic alliance, satisfaction with treatment, treatment completion, and symptom reduction. Bambling (2014) suggests that the mechanisms of change in supervision appear to be related not to the specific therapeutic approach but rather to common mechanisms. This notion is supported by Hill and Knox (2013) who argue that process factors such as the SR are important to achieve these outcomes although more work is needed to identify the specific mechanisms of change.

Bradshaw et al. (2007) conducted a study with 23 mental health nurses who were receiving supervision while working with 89 clients with a diagnosis of schizophrenia. Supervisors attended a two-day course in supervision. The nurses attended formal training (36 days) in psychosocial intervention and received small group clinical supervision. The experimental group also received regular fortnightly workplace clinical supervision in small groups. Outcome measures included measures of knowledge of case management and client symptom change. Both groups showed significant increases in knowledge and client improvement, but the supervisees who attended the additional workplace supervision group showed greater knowledge and their clients showed greater symptom reduction.

In another study with mental health nurses, E. White and Winstanley (2010) compared nurses who attended a monthly reflective supervision group for a year with those who did not receive supervision. Supervisors received four days of training in supervision skills. No difference was found between the supervised and unsupervised groups on a range of client outcome measures such as satisfaction and quality of care. While it was a carefully design using randomization, this study was conducted across a range of clinical sites with more nurses (186) than clients (170). Supervision groups were larger (six to nine members) and less frequent (monthly) than the previous studies discussed. The authors suggest that management issues across the various sites may have influenced the results. The type or quality of supervision provided and the quality of the SRs established are somewhat unclear but it appears likely, given the number of staff involved and the frequency of supervision sessions, that this would have been challenging to measure. This admirable study demonstrates some of the difficulties of conducting research that links client outcomes to supervision and, in particular, to the SR.

These three studies provide a promising direction in client outcome research in clinical supervision and raise a range of interesting questions for future practice and research. For example, how much training in supervision is sufficient to train an effective supervisor? What are the dosage effects? The Bambling et al. (2006) study involved weekly individual supervision, the Bradshaw et al. (2007) study fortnightly small groups, and in the E. White and Winstanley (2010) study larger groups of up to nine supervisees received monthly supervision. If the SR is a significant mutative factor, as the current research suggests, then what are the optimal conditions for it to develop? It is unlikely that the larger and less frequent groups supported strong development of the SR. The first two studies provided focused training and supervision on a particular therapeutic approach whereas the latter provided unstructured reflective groups. And, finally, there is a strong suggestion that contextual factors played a significant part in the outcomes of the White and Winstanley study, with variable support from management across the various sites in the study. This is interesting with the current contextual and service pressures (particularly in the National Health Service in the United Kingdom) to provide less frequent reflective group supervision. Currently, large, unstructured group supervision is contra-indicated by available research findings, although the evidence base is small.

A series of recent well-designed retrospective studies exploring client outcomes in a clinical psychology training clinic in the United States have shown significant effects for supervisor impact on client outcome (Callahan, Almstrom, Swift, Borja, & Heath, 2009), and the importance of supervisor competence and training on client outcomes, with more recently trained supervisors showing greater impact (Wrape, Callahan, Ruggero, & Watkins, 2015).

Outcome-Informed Practice

A major development in therapy research is the development of outcome-informed practice through session-by-session client feedback. Reese et al. (2009) explored the relationship between the SR, satisfaction with supervision, and client feedback in trainee therapists over a year. Trainees were divided into two groups, one receiving continuous client feedback from their supervisor and the other supervision as usual. Both supervision groups showed improved client outcomes but the client feedback group demonstrated significantly better outcomes. The SR and satisfaction with supervision was rated equally in both groups but supervisee self-efficacy was higher in the feedback condition. Grossl, Reese, Norsworthy, and Hopkins (2014), in a further study, explored whether the use of client session feedback led to differences in the SR, supervisee satisfaction, and client treatment outcome. Results indicated that supervisees who used session-by-session client feedback reported significantly higher satisfaction with supervision, but no differences were found between groups on supervisee ratings of the SR or client outcome. The authors suggest that these rather contradictory findings may be due to the small sample size, a lack of diversity, and a possible lack of adherence to the feedback condition. They argue that client feedback may be seen as more value-neutral (Worthen & Lambert, 2007) than supervisor feedback, and hence support a sense of collaboration within supervision that may impact on supervisee satisfaction. Swift et al. (2014) provide a useful discussion on how to effectively incorporate the use of objective client feedback into supervision discussions by exploring patterns of change as well as detailed discussion of specific clients.

Clinical case management (CCM) supervision is another method of outcome-informed supervision that has been developed for high-volume, low-intensity psychological interventions (Improving Access to Psychological Therapies [IAPT]) (Richards, 2014). It might be seen to best serve the fidelity, case management, and clinical governance functions of supervision. It involves the collection, collation, and feedback of routine clinical outcome measures and provides supervision alerts if treatment progress is not as expected. This method provides immediate and regular client feedback to supervisors and supervisees. CCM supervision is driven by two main factors: clinical outcomes and client engagement in treatment. Supervision involves detailed and regular case review and allows patterns to emerge and learning needs to be identified through the client outcome measures. CCM supervision is an organized and systematic approach that can provide a secure structure for supervisees, and has been found to be particularly useful for less experienced practitioners. The use of electronic systems of data collection provides an objective measurement of client progress. The supervision focus is on skills development, following a competency framework required by IAPT, ensuring adherence to the therapeutic model, and as such CCM fulfills mainly the normative functions of supervision. However, experienced supervisors may be able additionally to address the developmental and restorative aspects of supervision, if time and resources allow (Richards, 2014). It is unclear how CCM supervision impacts on the SR and, to our knowledge, little research has been conducted on the efficacy of this method of supervision. Although the IAPT program is clearly grounded in evidence-based methods of therapy, and supervision is very much part of the methodology (Turpin &Wheeler, 2011), little research has been conducted on how supervision supports this approach. Roth and Pilling (2008) suggest that there is an unquestioned assumption about the implicit benefit of supervision, which has resulted in therapy outcome trials often not measuring or detailing this important aspect of the work, rendering it "invisible" in research trails. Similarly, Milne et al. (2008) suggests that the lack of methodologically robust literature is particularly problematic in an area that prides itself on its underlying empiricism. Roth, Pilling, and Turner (2010) propose that one of the important aspects of supervision is to support adherence to treatment protocol. However, few studies have explored this. The Patton and Kivlighan (1997) study, discussed earlier, is important in this regard, suggesting that weekly fluctuations in the SR accounted for weekly fluctuations in following the treatment protocol in short-term psychodynamic therapy.

Measures of the Supervisory Relationship

The fundamental importance of the SR to successful supervision has been highlighted throughout the literature, but how do we assess the quality of our supervisory relationships? There are currently only a handful of measures of the SR, possibly reflecting the small number of models developed to explain its unique qualities. Those measures that have been developed have been criticized for their poor construction (Ellis et al., 2008). There is also some debate as to whether measures that have been directly imported from psychotherapy research are applicable in supervision research because of the very different nature of therapy and supervision, as identified in this book. There have been several reviews of outcome measures of supervision and the SR (Ellis & Ladany, 1997;

Ellis et al., 2008; Wheeler, Aveline, & Barkham, 2011). Those that attend specifically to the SR and are considered to meet acceptable psychometric standards are described in the sections that follow. These include the Relationship Inventory (Schacht, Howe, & Berman, 1989), the Working Alliance Inventory (Bahrick, 1990), and the Supervisory Working Alliance Inventory (Efstation et al., 1990). We shall then discuss the three measures of the SR that have been developed by the Oxford Supervision Research Group (OSRG), based on the models from our research. These include the Supervisory Relationship Questionnaire (SRQ) and its short form, the S-SRQ for supervisees, and the Supervisory Relationship Measure (SRM) for supervisors. A recent stringent review of measures of the SR (Tangen & Borders, 2016, p. 177) suggests that "At this point, the SRQ, S-SRQ, and SRM seem especially exhaustive in investigations of validity and reliability and thus may be the most viable choices for researchers and practitioners with regard to construction criteria."

The Relationship Inventory (RI)

The RI (Schacht et al., 1988) is a measure of the SR based on the "facilitative conditions" for therapeutic change within humanistic models. It is a rating scale composed of five subscales measuring perceived supervisor relational qualities, namely regard, empathy, congruence, unconditionality, and willingness to be known. The inventory was originally developed to measure the therapeutic relationship (the Barrett-Lennard Relationship Inventory: Barrett-Lennard, 1962). It was adapted for use in supervision by changing some of the wording, for example replacing "therapist" with "supervisor." It was validated using a sample of clinical and counseling psychologists in the United States and is considered to have acceptable psychometric properties.

The Working Alliance Inventory (WAI)

The WAI (Bahrick, 1990) was developed to test Bordin's (1983) model of the Supervisory Working Alliance (SWA), based on his model of the therapeutic alliance. Similar to the RI measure, the WAI was adapted from a measure originally designed to assess the therapeutic alliance. It measures the three components of the SWA, namely, the degree of agreement on the goals of supervision, the tasks to be completed, and the bond that develops between supervisee and supervisor. The WAI has parallel trainee and supervisor versions and has good psychometric properties. Ellis et al. (2008) argue that the three factors (goals, tasks, and bond) are highly correlated and hence suggest the WAI may be measuring a single alliance factor.

The Supervisory Working Alliance Inventory (SWAI)

The SWAI (Efstation et al., 1990) is another widely used measure of the SR. The SWAI is derived from both psychotherapy and supervision models and has non-parallel supervisor and supervisee versions. The supervisor version comprises three factors: client focus, rapport, and identification. The supervisee version comprises two factors: rapport and client focus. Low internal consistency has been reported. There is some debate in the literature as to its psychometric properties, with Wheeler et al. (2011), in their review of measures, recommending its use and Ellis and Ladany (1997) questioning its psychometric robustness.

The Brief Supervisory Alliance Scale—trainee form (BSAS-TF)

The BSAS-TF (Rønnestad and Lundquist, 2009) is also recommended by Wheeler et al. (2011) in their review. This measure is considered to have acceptable psychometric properties and is recommended for its brevity (12 items). Unfortunately, it is not widely available as it is unpublished, but it is available from the authors.

The Role Conflict and Role Ambiguity Scale (RCRA)

The RCRA (Olk & Friedlander, 1992) is another interesting measure that has been widely used in supervision research and has good psychometric properties. Although the RCRA is not a measure of the SR per se, it is useful in identifying some of the issues that may contribute to strains in the SR such as a supervisee's lack of clarity regarding role expectations.

All the published measures of the SR described in this chapter have normative data drawn from US populations (of counselors, psychotherapists, clinical and counseling psychologists). They have been widely used in research, predominantly in training settings. Several of the measures are direct adaptations of measures of the therapeutic relationship and hence may not fully assess the unique aspects of the SR. In particular, the educative, evaluative, and involuntary nature of many training SRs may not be captured by the measures discussed thus far. Additionally, there may be elements of service and of the professional and national culture that are specific to measures drawn largely from North America, which are not applicable to training, service, or cultural contexts elsewhere.

In the next section, we describe the measures that we have developed to address some of the issues and gaps identified in the literature, psychometrically robust outcome measures that specifically measure the unique features of the SR.

Measures of the Supervisory Relationship Developed by the Oxford Supervision Research Group (OSRG)

Three measures, based on qualitative research on the SR, have been developed by the OSRG: the SRQ and the S-SRQ for supervisees, and the SRM for supervisors. These will be discussed in detail here and are included in the appendices. The SRQ, S-SRQ, and SRM were developed with UK samples of trainee and qualified psychologists working in the National Health Service.

The Supervisory Relationship Questionnaire (SRQ)

Palomo (2004) used the qualitative model developed by Beinart (2002; described in Chapter 2) to develop a psychometrically sound measure of the SR from the supervisees' perspective. This is known as the Supervisory Relationship Questionnaire (Palomo et al., 2010; see Appendix 1). Exploratory factor analysis was used to analyze the responses from 284 trainee clinical psychologists to develop a valid and reliable measure of the SR, as well as to explore perceived impacts on client outcome and supervisee learning and development. The SRQ has 67 items and good psychometric properties. The analysis yielded six coherent factors: (a) safe base; (b) structure; (c) commitment; (d) reflective education; (e) role model; and (f) formative feedback. The components reflect the distinct nature of the supervisory relationship, including its educative, involuntary, and evaluative nature, as well as its central core component, the "safe base," which reflects the more generic facilitative, relational characteristics. The safe base factor was found to be the strongest predictor of supervisee-rated outcome measures of learning and development and client outcomes. Milne (2009) has used the factors from the SRQ to develop suggestions for improving supervisory practice. These include the importance of establishing an emotional connection, sharing expectations, providing regular and structured supervision, being approachable and attentive, showing respect for clients and colleagues, encouraging reflection, and providing regular and balanced feedback. The SRQ has also been widely incorporated into supervisor training programs in the United Kingdom (Fleming & Steen, 2013) and is increasingly used in international research as a robust outcome measure.

The Short Supervisory Relationship Questionnaire (S-SRQ)

The SRQ, although psychometrically and theoretically robust, has been criticized for being too lengthy for day-to-day clinical practice (Wheeler et al., 2011). In a recent study (Cliffe, Beinart, & Cooper, 2014) developed a short version of the SRQ, the S-SRQ (see Appendix 2). Two hundred and three UK trainee clinical psychologists completed a series of online questionnaires including the S-SRQ. A principal components analysis identified three components of the S-SRQ: safe base; reflective education; and structure. Analyses revealed that the S-SRQ has high internal reliability, adequate test–retest reliability, and good convergent, divergent, criterion, and predictive validity. Participants also rated the S-SRQ as easy to use and potentially helpful for providing feedback on the SR within supervision. The S-SRQ (three subscales, with a total of 18 items) is a short, easy-to-use, valid, and reliable measure of the supervisory relationship from the supervisee's perspective (Cliffe et al., 2014).

The Supervisory Relationship Measure (SRM)

Pearce et al. (2013) used the qualitative findings and model of the SR developed by Clohessy (2008, described in Chapter 2) to develop a questionnaire, the Supervisory Relationship Measure, to assess the SR from the perspective of the supervisor (see Appendix 3). Exploratory factor analysis was used to analyze the data from 267 clinical psychology supervisors. The results suggested a five-factor structure: (a) safe base; (b) supervisor commitment; (c) trainee contribution; (d) external influences; and (e) supervisor investment. The SRM has good psychometric properties including acceptable levels of internal consistency, good convergent and divergent validity, and high levels of retest reliability. The SRM also shows promise as a useful statistical predictor of trainee competence (as perceived by the supervisor) and supervisor satisfaction with supervision.

Aspects of Clohessy's model, such as the core relational factors, are reflected in the safe base and supervisor investment subscales. The concept of the "flow of supervision" can be seen in the trainee contribution, supervisor commitment, and safe base subscales. The contextual factors are represented in the external influences subscale. As with its sister measure, the SRQ, safe base appeared to be the strongest predictor of supervision outcomes, including perceived effectiveness, lending strong support to the supervisory working alliance being an important component of the SR. However, the SRM also affirms the influence of contextual factors and supervisee contribution, and confirms the hypotheses that, while there are common elements to the SR, supervisors and supervisees may have somewhat different views and experiences of their SRs. Some implications for practice for supervisees, supervisors, and the supervisory dyad based on the SRM factors have emerged. These include being open and honest, demonstrating enthusiasm and commitment, and taking a personal interest in the unique characteristics of the supervisee.

The measures have the advantage of being psychometrically sound and of being based explicitly on supervision theory and research. They also provide a good choice for those seeking measures based within a UK as opposed to a US health-care system and have recently been recommended for use in research and practice (Tangen & Borders, 2016).

Session-by-Session Measures of the Supervisory Relationship

An interesting recent development in the field of measuring the SR is the Leeds Alliance in Supervision Scale (LASS), a three-item scale designed to provide session-by-session feedback on the supervisory alliance. It consists of three visual analog scales: approach to supervision, the relationship, and the degree to which the supervisee found supervision helpful. It is based on measures of the SR and is reported to have acceptable levels of validity and reliability, and, importantly, it is sensitive to change (Wainwright, 2010).

Summary

We have looked at the various outcomes in supervision and attempted to distil the research on the impact of the SR on supervision outcomes related to both the supervisees' learning and experience of supervision, as well as exploring the few studies that have looked at client outcome. We have introduced the emerging area of outcome-informed practice and discussed some of the research in this developing area. We have also described some of the more methodologically sound measures that assess the SR, including the three developed by our research group. These are included in the appendices of this volume. Bernard and Goodyear (2014), in their most recent edition, suggest that all the processes in supervision are mediated by the SR and this appears to be born out by the evidence. Much work is still needed on the mechanisms involved in this process and, in particular, on how the SR influences the experiences of supervisees and clients in the different contexts they practice. We need to bear in mind that much of the current research has been conducted in counseling or psychology training contexts in the United States with the addition of some important studies from Australia and the United Kingdom. This may not reflect the experiences of supervisees and their clients working in other contexts. For example, Son, Ellis, and Yoo (2013) found that the relationship between working alliance and satisfaction was stronger for American compared to Korean supervisees. We need to bear in mind the context of the research and that findings may not be transferable across contexts. In the next chapter we shall discuss the influence of values, culture, and ethics on the SR.

Key Points

- Assessing outcome in supervision is complex and challenging.
- The supervisory relationship is pivotal to effective supervision and there are a number of psychometrically robust measures available. These can be used in research contexts and also in supervisory practice to review the relationship.
- Outcomes in supervision can be defined in multiple ways, including the impact of supervision on the supervisee (satisfaction with supervision, changes in supervisee knowledge and skills, self-efficacy, and well-being) and positive client change.
- Attending to session-by-session client outcome measures in supervision may be one way of focusing and structuring supervision and of explicitly attending to client outcomes.

5

Ethical and Culturally Sensitive Practice

The aims of this chapter are:

- to consider the impact and influence of values, ethics, and ethical decision-making;
- to explore the role of culture and diversity in the supervisory relationship.

As we have discussed in Chapter 3, the supervisory relationship has multiple influences. In this chapter, we shall focus on some of these influences in more detail, including values, ethics, culture, context, and diversity. Underpinning issues such as ethical and culturally sensitive practice is the concept of values. In the United Kingdom, values-based practice in mental health has been promoted as a partner to the more familiar evidence-based practice. Values include the unique preferences, concerns, and expectations each person brings to an encounter. The recognition that each individual contributes a unique set of values underpins ethical and diversity-sensitive practice. It has also formed the basis of a number of national and international policy, training, and service development initiatives (e.g., Fulford, 2008; Woodbridge & Fulford, 2004). Values-based practice aims to provide a framework for enabling people to work in a respectful and sensitive manner with an appreciation of the different values they may encounter in their work (Woodbridge & Fulford, 2004). There is a close association between values and ethics but values can be seen as a broader concept. For example, values underpin ethical decision-making, which may include personal preferences, and are likely to be influenced by broader cultural factors such as religious or political beliefs. Values are also likely to be influenced by historical time; for example, attitudes to gender and to same-sex relationships have changed significantly over the past half-century. Values may also underpin attitudes to power. For example, individuals raised in more collectivist cultures may value the authority of experience and position more highly than those from more individualist cultures (Tsui, O'Donoghue, & Ng, 2014). Similarly, individuals may place different emphases on the importance of core relational variables such as honesty, trust, and respect. Values-based practice lends itself well to a systemic approach that privileges multiple perspectives (see Chapter 2). It assumes that the individual exists within a number of social systems and has different roles and social identities within each of them (e.g., partner, parent, worker, friend, supervisor). It helps us move away from a

Effective Supervisory Relationships: Best Evidence and Practice, First Edition.
Helen Beinart and Sue Clohessy.
© 2017 John Wiley & Sons Ltd. Published 2017 by John Wiley & Sons Ltd.

problem focus to a more person-centered approach that recognizes the uniqueness of the individual. It also requires the practitioner to engage in reflective practice, particularly when they come across values that conflict with their own (see Chapter 9). The approach is not to debate right and wrong but to respect and explore the differences and their influences with the aim to reach a more in depth understanding. Additionally, Tervalon and Murray-Garcia (1998) suggest adopting a position of cultural humility that involves a lifelong commitment to self-evaluation and critique, addressing power dynamics and developing mutually beneficial partnerships. Value-based practice and cultural humility are both useful meta-concepts that underpin sound SRs (Watkins & Hook, 2016). The starting point in any SR is to recognize and to remain aware of, and sensitive and open to, the unique values and perspectives in the room. Not only is this a good point from which to begin to negotiate a working relationship, but it also provides a helpful model for relating to others (whether clients or staff) in an ethical way that is likely to value their unique perspectives and remain sensitive to difference.

Ethics in Supervision and the Supervisory Relationship

One of the key tasks of supervision, particularly for those early in their careers, is socialization into the ethics of a profession and integration of ethics into professional behavior. The SR provides a unique opportunity for the supervisor to model ethical behavior and to discuss the values that underpin professional ethical practice. An ethical stance within the SR values the dignity of others, responsible caring, transparency, engagement, attentiveness, as well as humility, flexibility, and professionalism (Falender, Burnes, & Ellis, 2013). The SR provides the forum for these discussions and the quality of the SR is likely to impact the quality of learning. The negotiation of power and involvement (Holloway, 1995; see Chapter 2) is central to developing a collaborative relationship that enhances the supervisee's learning while maintaining the welfare of the client as paramount. Similarly, developing a supervisory contract is a key task of developing a SR where both parties are aware of the expectations, responsibilities, and limits of their roles. This would include ethical obligations such as the primacy of the service user, the management of power, and professional gatekeeping functions.

Although there is not scope here for a full analysis of power within the SR, it is worth mentioning the early model proposed by French and Raven (1959) regarding social power which, applied to supervision, is still a helpful way to explain how supervisors may use their power for the benefit or to the detriment of the SR. French and Raven refer to:

- reward power, where the supervisor mediates rewards;
- coercive power, where the supervisor mediates punishments;
- legitimate power, where the supervisor has legitimate authority;
- referent power, where the supervisee identifies with supervisor;
- expert power, which is based on the supervisor's knowledge and skills.

Although the supervisor has hierarchical power within the SR (which may incorporate all aspects of power described), both supervisors and supervisees are responsible for adhering to ethical guidelines. Therefore, behaving ethically within the SR is a shared responsibility. A strong ethical framework supports an effective and mutually respectful SR, which enhances learning, which in turn results in enhanced performance and protects all those affected by the work, including students, clients, research participants, supervisees, and supervisors (Pettifor, McCarron, Schoepp, Stark, & Stewart, 2011).

Principles of beneficence, non-maleficence, respect for autonomy, justice, and fairness underpin most international ethical codes. In the United Kingdom, the Code of Ethics and Conduct for psychology (British Psychological Society [BPS], 2009) includes the principles of respect, competence, responsibility, and integrity. Professional ethical codes generally provide a basis for decision-making and for regulating the professions. As such, they provide a contract with society about acceptable professional behavior. Internationally, supervisors may face similar ethical issues in their SRs, including boundaries and multiple relationships, competence, due process, informed consent, confidentiality, and multicultural competence. These key areas are discussed in more detail in the sections that follow.

Ethical Issues within the Supervisory Relationship

Boundaries and Multiple Relationships

Multiple relationships in supervision occur when the supervisor and supervisee have more than one social role in relation to one another. These are common and not necessarily unethical. For example, a supervisee may also act as a research assistant for their supervisor. Changes in role over time are also common. For example, a previous trainee may join a staff team and become a colleague, and potentially a friend. However, multiple relationships can become problematic if there is a misuse of power and the person with less power is at risk of exploitation (Bernard & Goodyear, 2014). Supervisors need to be mindful of the issue of multiple relationships when supervising their supervisee's working relationships with their clients. A typical example of misuse of power is where supervisees engage in inappropriate relationships with their clients—ranging from a friendship to a sexual relationship. The same is true for the SR. Developing a more personal relationship with a supervisee can be problematic. For example, if the supervisor befriends the supervisee, it may be difficult to raise concerns about supervisee competence. This is a tricky balance for supervisors to maintain—they need to develop enough safety within the SR for the supervisee to disclose personal information that is relevant to their work. A certain level of familiarity is needed for the SR to work effectively but boundaries also need to be made explicit, firm, and clear. This is not always the case; Ladany, Mori, and Mehr (2013) found that most of the supervisory transgressions in their study concerned boundary infringements. It is not uncommon for feelings of personal or sexual attraction to enter the SR. Some studies (e.g., Rodolfa et al., 1994) suggest that a quarter of interns in postdoctoral internship sites reported feeling sexual attraction toward their clinical supervisor. Ladany, Friedlander, and Nelson (2005) argue that these possibilities should be introduced as part of early negotiations within the SR in order to normalize them. They encourage supervisors to note any markers of potential boundary vulnerability both with clients and within the SR. These may include verbal markers (e.g., expression of strong feelings) and non-verbal markers (e.g., change in appearance). Bernard and Goodyear (2014) advise the use of a professional disclosure statement during contracting (see Chapter 6) to act as a deterrent to boundary violation. Such a statement includes information about the supervisor's training (including training in supervision) and experience, issues of confidentiality, and contact information for an external adviser should there be any concerns within the SR. They suggest that this communicates high regard for professionalism and integrity. Several authors advocate the use of supplementary supervisory arrangements such as peer or group supervision to help reduce the risk of boundary infringements.

Multiple relationships are a broad category and cover a wide continuum, either end of which is relatively clear. There is, however, a broad middle ground of potential ethical complexity if supervisors and supervisees engage in multiple relationships.

Competence

Competence frameworks for supervision have been developed in various countries, including the United Kingdom (CORE guidance; Roth & Pilling, 2008), the Psychology Board of Australia (2013), and more recently the American Psychological Association (APA; Guidelines for Clinical Supervision in Health Service Psychology: American Psychological Association, 2015). In addition to the development of these national frameworks and guidelines, some authors are working toward international competency benchmarks for clinical supervision (Olds & Hawkins, 2014; see Chapter 1).

Supervisor competence is the core of all these guidelines as well as being a core ethical requirement for professional practice (e.g., BPS Code of Ethics and Conduct: BPS, 2009). There are two broad areas of supervisor competence: professional competence in the area being supervised and knowledge and skills in supervision itself. It is important to recognize that supervision is a distinct professional activity with knowledge, skills, and attitudes that require specific training (Falender, Burnes, & Ellis, 2013). Supervisors are also in the position of having to assess the competence of their supervisees, particularly during training. Historically, it has been assumed that clinical or professional competence bestows on an individual the ability to supervise. This may be the case for the competence in the area being supervised but it is no longer acceptable for competence in supervision itself. The growing competency movement within supervision (e.g., Falender et al., 2013) argues persuasively that supervision has its own set of competencies that require training and development.

Ladany (2014) has written comprehensively about poor supervision and suggests that about a third of all SRs are weak, a third adequate, and a third effective.

Ellis et al. (2014), in their careful study of inadequate and harmful supervision, found that over 90% of supervisees reported that they had received inadequate supervision and 35% reported harmful supervision. Additionally, over half of their participants reported harmful supervision at some point in their careers. We have to conclude from these findings that competence in supervision is a major ethical issue that needs to be addressed.

It is reasonable to assume that the majority of practitioners who qualify are competent at the point of qualification (if supervisors are competently fulfilling their gate-keeping role). However, competence is not static and needs to be continually updated and refreshed. It is an ethical obligation to refresh and develop practice skills. The same is true for supervisory knowledge and skills. A once-off attendance at an introductory supervisor training course is not sufficient training for an entire supervisory career, particularly if supervision practice is intermittent. The American Psychological Association (2015, p. 36) guidance states that,

> at a minimum, education and training in supervision should include the following: models and theories of supervision; modalities; relationship formation, maintenance rupture and repair; diversity and multiculturalism; feedback, evaluation; management of supervisee's emotional reactivity and interpersonal behaviour; reflective practice; application of ethical and legal standards; decision making regarding gatekeeping; and consideration of the developmental level of the trainee.

Additionally, competence should be informed by evidence-based practice, up-to-date research, the use of current measures (Milne & Reiser, 2012), and feedback. A core function of supervision is to develop and monitor supervisee competence. However, one of the most challenging aspects of supervision, particularly for new supervisors, is the evaluative and gate-keeping role. This is particularly challenging if the consequences for the supervisee are failing a training program. However, it is a supervisor's core ethical responsibility to gate-keep for their profession. It is also normative for supervisors to experience gate-keeping anxiety (M. L. Nelson, Barnes, Evans, & Triggiano, 2008). There is a danger of the "cult of the positive" (Brown & Marzillier, 1993) and, if supervisees are in training, a risk of leniency or lack of responsibility, in letting the next supervisor pick up and address any problematic issues. The balance between supporting development and evaluating competency is a difficult one and supervisors need to make complex and challenging judgments in this area. The area of assessment, evaluation, and feedback is an essential component of ethical supervision, and formative feedback is key to managing this process. The reader is referred to Chapter 7 on feedback for a full discussion on managing this process effectively.

Due Process

Due process relates to the gate-keeping function of supervision and ensures that supervisees are competent. Due process is a particular ethical issue for supervisors who are concerned with training the next generation of their profession as well as those who supervise for registration bodies post-qualification. It involves the ethical principles of fairness and equality. Due process has two components, sometimes referred to as *substantive* and *procedural.* Substantive due process refers to whether the substance of a decision is fair rather than arbitrary. Procedural due process concerns the individual's right to be notified of any requirements and regulations, to be made aware if they are not meeting these, and to receive regular feedback and evaluation (Thomas, 2010). The standards for counseling supervisors (Dye & Borders, 2011) state clearly that supervisors should attend to the principles of informed consent and due process within their institutions, training programs, and individual SRs. The most frequently cited example of due process infringement occurs when a supervisee is failed from a training program or dismissed from a job without being given feedback or prior warning that they were not meeting the expectations required of them, or provided with the opportunity to improve their performance. In such cases, supervisees may decide to appeal and, if the supervisor has not followed due process procedures, it is likely that the decision will be seen as unfair and not supported by the institution. This situation can have very unfortunate personal and professional consequences and may involve multiple other ethical infringements including issues of confidentiality, informed consent, and competence.

The implications of due process for the SR include ensuring that a relationship is established and maintained where expectations are clear and supervisees are given regular feedback on their development and skill progression, and the opportunity to address any areas of concern. Supervisors should also ensure that they follow relevant due process procedures, and that they seek their own supervision and guidance to ensure that their decisions are fair and equitable.

Informed Consent

Professional ethical codes all discuss the importance of obtaining informed consent from clients. However, many are silent on how this should be applied in supervision. Informed client consent would usually include a discussion of the risks and benefits of an intervention, identify alternatives, discuss limits to confidentiality, and explain reporting obligations. The ethical task is to assist the client in making an informed choice by providing sufficient information to allow them to make a reasonable decision. The person must be competent to make the choice, which is generally voluntary, without any undue influence or coercion.

These principles apply only partly to supervision where, at least during training, there is a requirement to participate in supervision and there may be a limited choice of supervisors. It is assumed that an informed choice occurs when trainees apply to a particular training program. Once accepted, they have to comply with certain parameters (Thomas, 2010). These include the learning outcomes or competencies required, the process of evaluation, and mandatory supervision.

However, it is strongly recommended that, within these restricted parameters of consent, informed consent is sought from supervisees (Bernard & Goodyear, 2014; Thomas, 2010). Cobia and Boes (2000) argue that truly informed consent, one that includes a professional disclosure statement and formal plans for supervision, enhances the SR and creates a collaborative environment for learning. As an important part of developing the supervision contract, it also provides the opportunity to clarify goals, structures, methods, and the overall purpose of supervision. It is an effective way of establishing boundaries and accountability, and of reducing the risk of misunderstanding (see Chapter 6 for further discussion on contracting).

Confidentiality

Confidentiality is the most common supervisory ethical problem cited by psychologists internationally, as well as the most common boundary infringement reported in the United States (Pettifor & Sawchuck, 2006). Confidentiality is defined as a professional obligation not to disclose information unless agreed by the individual(s) concerned. It is an obligation or promise regarding a contract between two parties, but it is not a formal legal contract. Practitioners are often required to make a decision about whether it is in the client's best interest to disclose information where their privacy or confidentiality is compromised. Professionals will often have to weigh up other ethical or legal considerations, bearing in mind that the welfare of the client is paramount.

Similar to the many other variables discussed in relation to supervision, confidentiality is a multilayered phenomenon and concerns both supervisee information and disclosures, and information pertaining to the client and their context.

Supervisee Confidentiality

Ladany and Lehrman-Waterman (1999) reported that supervisor–supervisee confidentiality was one of the most common ethical issues encountered in their study. However, professional ethical codes provide little guidance on supervisee disclosure, which is not typically considered confidential because of the gatekeeping function of supervision. This is a challenging issue for the SR that needs to be managed transparently and sensitively. Practitioners recognize that personal factors (e.g., values, beliefs, experience) influence their capacity to understand and relate to their clients, and on the whole make them more empathic and responsive. However, at times work issues can interact with personal issues and lead to heightened emotional reactivity, which may reduce their capacity to empathize with the client (Falender, Shafranske, & Falicov, 2014). As professionals develop, they develop an understanding of the more personal aspects of their work (often through personal therapy, reflective practice, and good supervision). Competent practitioners learn to watch out for, and to work with, any personal resonances and reactivity. Exploration of these issues is appropriate material for supervision and needs to be managed sensitively and constructively by maintaining a focus on the best interests of the client. On occasion, a supervisor may advise that the supervisee seek counseling or therapy if there are unresolved personal issues that need further exploration. However, in evaluative SRs, this material may potentially be shared with others in the training institution or management structure, particularly if a supervisor is concerned about supervisee welfare or performance. A conversation regarding the limits of confidentiality needs to take place in the contracting phase of supervision so that the supervisee can make an informed choice about the personal material they choose to share in supervision. Nevertheless, it is good practice for a supervisor who feels they need to discuss the supervisee's personal disclosures outside of the SR, to inform the supervisee and seek their consent. For example, a supervisor may note that a supervisee appears to be struggling with a particular aspect of their work, and may want to find out from colleagues if this has been a pattern throughout training or is relevant only to a particular working context or client group. This would be a useful conversation to have with the supervisee in the first instance, and it would demonstrate an openness and transparency that is likely to strengthen the SR. However, these are sensitive and potentially difficult ethical dilemmas that should be handled with care and respect. Indeed, in a recent study Pakdaman, Shafranske, and Falender (2014) explored ethical issues within SRs and confirmed previous findings that it was the strength of the relationship that influenced the degree of disclosure offered.

Confidentiality Concerning Others

This is an area that is fully covered in all professional ethical guidance. It is clear that client information must be kept confidential, with some caveats normally involving safeguarding and client welfare. However, supervision itself is a third-party discussion, and supervisors may receive their own supervision and, in certain contexts, discussion within a team working with the client may be considered best practice. Confidentiality within the SR is multilayered and complex, and needs sensitive and transparent handling. The situation becomes even more complex in group supervision where it is essential that clear ground rules be established regarding confidentiality and anonymity. Similarly, the use of supervision recordings, and technology such as email or Skype, to support supervision adds its own confidentiality dimension that needs to be carefully considered and appropriate safety measures need to be put in place. It may be that professional guidelines need to be updated to cover these newer methods of supervision. The reader is referred to Rousmaniere (2014) on the use of technology in supervision for a full discussion of ethical issues posed by new technologies.

Ethical Decision-Making

The SR provides the cornerstone of ethical decision-making by modeling best practice in this regard. It brings us back to the teaching of values-based practice raised earlier in this chapter. Some authors have referred to this as developing moral expertise (Narvaez & Lapsley, 2005). Ethical decision-making often starts with considering personal values that may be influenced by a range of cultural factors such as familial, political, or religious beliefs. All training programs teach ethical codes but few practitioners appear to apply these consciously when grappling with complex ethical decisions. This may be because they are so ingrained that they have become automatic but it is important that every professional, particularly a supervisor, is able to draw explicitly on the relevant ethical code and to use it to guide their supervisees. Supervision provides a safe space to explore ethical dilemmas and practice and to apply ethical knowledge. Supervisors can utilize their power to model best practice by being explicit about their values, using ethical codes and openly grappling with complex decisions that are an inevitable part of their work. Although there are many commonalities between the ethical codes of different professional groups, each profession has slightly different emphases, and professional ethics is often a way of acclimatizing a new member to a particular professional culture. Supervision provides the opportunity for this ethical "acculturation" to a particular profession through discussion of overarching ethical values, principles, and rules.

Traditionally ethical principles and ethical decision-making have been taught as a structured process. For example, many professional groups use the four levels of ethical decision-making identified by Beauchamp and Childress (1994; 2013), which suggest that there should be a discussion of the following:

- philosophical or theoretical position: the governing assumptive worldview of the client, supervisee, and supervisor, and wider contexts;
- ethical principles relevant to the issue, for example, confidentiality, beneficence;
- rules and expectations relevant to the issue, for example, a code of ethics and conduct;
- action required, for example, seeking informed consent.

More recently, in an attempt to ensure that supervision addresses the complexity of professional ethics in a multicultural society, the behavioral expectations or rules aspect of ethical decision-making has been challenged (Pettifor, Sinclair, & Falender, 2014). These authors raise the complexity of working in settings where clients, supervisees, and supervisors may have differing cultural values, expectations, and worldviews, and stress the importance of responding to cultural difference within supervision. They suggest an ideal process whereby the SR is based on cultural humility and a respectful collaborative process in which "the supervisory expectations are clearly delineated; the effect of the world views of the supervisor, supervisee, and client are addressed; and all parties are treated with respect and fairness" (Pettifor et al., 2014, p. 202). In this way, the focus of ethical decision-making is seen as more values-based and individualized to a particular supervisory dyad and client need, rather than following a set of prescribed rules and structures that may have been developed from a different value base (this is discussed in the next section).

International Perspectives

Ethical codes are shaped by social, political, legal, economic, and cultural contexts (Thomas, 2014; Tsui, O'Donoghue, & Ng, 2014). Western codes tend to emphasize the individual, personal autonomy, and boundaries. Conversely, some cultures emphasize community, family, and interdependence between people. In these contexts, some Western ethical standards may not be fully applicable, for example, the importance of professional boundaries and objectivity, the balance of independence and autonomous decision-making, and perceived responsibilities to family and community. In response to these differences, there has been an effort in recent years to develop international ethics codes (Gauthier & Pettifor, 2012). The Universal Declaration of Ethical Principles for Psychologists (Gauthier, 2008) is based on four ethical principles:

- respect for the dignity of persons and peoples;
- competent caring for the well-being of persons and peoples;
- integrity;
- professional and scientific responsibilities to society.

It seems that it is somewhat easier to agree on international principles and ideals than on specific behavioral rules and standards, which appear to be more culturally differentiated, and most countries prefer to have their own specific standards and quality control mechanisms (Gauthier & Pettifor, 2012).

This intersection between ethics and culture within the SR and the importance of cultural humility, sensitivity to diversity, and cultural competence within the relationship between supervisor and supervisee will be discussed in more detail in the next section.

Diversity and Cultural Competence

Our changing multicultural society has shifted thinking in this area enormously over the past half-century, and professional guidance has not always kept up with the pace of change. It is now common for practitioners from different backgrounds and cultures to be trained and/or to practice in a country different from their country of origin. Migration has also lead to an increased likelihood that supervisors, supervisees, and clients will come from various cultures. Inga-Britt Krause (1998, p. 4) defines culture as "a social construction created, maintained, reconstituted and changed through social relationships both public and private, general and intimate." Vargas, Porter, and Falender (2008, p. 122) provide a more detailed definition: "the dynamic and active process of constructing shared meaning, as represented by shared ideas, beliefs, attitudes, values, norms, practices, language, spirituality, and symbols, with acknowledgement and consideration of positions of power, privilege, and oppression."

The SR has to be open, flexible, and inclusive enough to incorporate multiple cultures and values, both within the relationship between supervisor and supervisee, and in relation to the work of the supervisee with their clients. The term "cultural competence" began to appear in the supervision literature in the 1990s and is now incorporated into most professional codes. In this section, "culture" is used as a collective term to cover all forms of diversity, including race, ethnicity, gender, sexual orientation, and spirituality. The work of John Burnham (2011) and colleagues is helpful in this context. They refer to numerous aspects of difference using the acronym "Social Graces." Over time, these "graces" have extended (and continue to grow) to cover numerous aspects of diversity—gender, geography, race, religion, age, ability, appearance, class, culture, education, ethnicity, employment, sexuality, sexual orientation, and spirituality (GGRRAAACCEEESSS). This helpful tool allows us to acknowledge and name differences, and provides a means of exploration of difference within the SR (discussed in Chapter 9).

When discussing cultural variations, the terms "etic" (outsider) and "emic" (insider) are often used. Those adhering to an etic stance often hold a universalist position by focusing on what they believe is universal and common in human nature at the expense of recognizing culturally normative differences. An emic position aims to understand difference from the inside by taking an empathic stance and attempting to understand the world through the perspective of the other. This means maintaining an interest, openness, and curiosity to hearing and learning about other experiences. In supervision this cannot take place without an open and trusting SR.

Most definitions of multicultural competence in supervision stem from the early work of D. W. Sue, Arredondo, and McDavis (1992), which focused on multicultural knowledge and skills. More recently, the emphasis has shifted to values and attitudes, as well as incorporating broader ideas regarding diversity and social justice (Falender et al., 2014).

Models and Research Relating to Cultural Competence in Supervision

In order to develop cultural competence, Bernard and Goodyear (2014) suggest that supervisors attend to four dimensions:

- intrapersonal identity (e.g., racial, gender, sexual, class identities that affect a person's sense of self);
- interpersonal biases (e.g., prejudices toward another based on membership of a particular group);
- interpersonal cultural identity and behavior (e.g., understanding of normative social role behaviors);
- sociopolitical influences (e.g., the level of privilege or power a person experiences on a range of cultural dimensions such as race and gender).

This involves supervisors developing an increased understanding and awareness of their *own* cultural backgrounds including those that may be members of dominant cultures. There are several models for the development of cultural competence. For example, D. Sue and D. W. Sue (2008) propose a model comprising the following stages:

- conformity (prior to reflection);
- dissonance (self-doubt);
- resistance (immersion in identity);
- introspection;
- integrative awareness (e.g., of racial, religious, cultural, sexual, professional identities with personal identity).

As well as understanding their own cultural background, supervisors also need to develop an increased knowledge and understanding of different cultures that may be represented by their supervisees or clients. In a multicultural context, this may be seen as a daunting task, but a safe and trusting SR provides the opportunity for a dialogue about cultural differences and power within supervision. A stance of cultural humility can greatly enhance these explorations (Falender & Shafranske, 2012). The supervisor also has the task of supporting the supervisee's cultural competence through modeling cultural sensitivity and encouraging collaborative discussions in supervision (Tsui et al., 2014).

Living in a multicultural society makes the complex issue of cultural variables in supervision both important and challenging. For example, a particular behavior or communication may have quite different meanings and consequences in different cultures and therefore an appropriate response in one culture may not be appropriate in another. Our experience in clinical psychology training in the United Kingdom is that many SRs act as if they are culturally "blind" and take the position that they will deal with difference and diversity only if it becomes a problem. This perspective may be due to the supervisor taking a "universalist" position (i.e., we are all the same) or to bias, lack of awareness, or uncertainty about how to talk about culture. However, within the SR, if cultural differences are not addressed, the potential for strain or rupture within the SR is likely to be increased, not least since the supervisee may feel misunderstood. Additionally, the power of the supervisor may be amplified by privilege of position, education, and socioeconomic status (Falender et al., 2014).

The limited research in this area suggests that most practitioners consider themselves culturally competent, but specific cultural practices do not support that belief (Hansen et al., 2006). Findings suggest that supervisors believe that they introduce discussion of diversity and difference in supervision. However, supervisees report that, if the subject comes up at all, they are the ones who raise it and that their initiative is not always well received or accepted (Jernigan, Green, Helms, Perez-Gualdron, & Henze, 2010). Generational differences, and the value attached to multiculturalism, are possible explanations for the supervisor–supervisee mismatch in this area. It is often those whose cultures appear to represent the dominant values within a particular society who see no need to explore the complexity of culture and cultural identity and thus may unquestioningly accept culturally determined values, thereby losing a rich potential strand of learning.

Burnham and Harris (2002) suggest that it is helpful to consider three interlinked domains when considering how culture impacts supervision. These are summarized in Table 5.1. Burnham (2011) highlights a helpful way of approaching diversity in supervision and invites us to consider that social differences may vary between being visible and voiced (e.g., gender); visible and unvoiced (e.g., age); invisible and voiced (e.g., class); and invisible and unvoiced (e.g., spirituality). He notes that we all have a tendency to privilege aspects of diversity that hold meaning for us and often ignore others, potential blind spots that could be helpful to explore (see Chapter 9 for reflective practice exercises).

Practitioners tend to privilege their preferred areas (where they feel more competent or about which they are more passionate) and may subjugate other areas they consider outside their comfort zone, often without noticing. Burnham's

Table 5.1 Domains of cultural influence on supervision (Burnham & Harris, 2002).

Domain	Examples
Culture of supervisory practice	Professional or training context Theoretical influences Modality Value of supervision within working context
Culture within the SR	Similarities and differences between supervisor and supervisee Openness to discussion about values Willingness to explore power
Culture within practice relationships	Similarities and differences between practitioner and clients Ability to be open and to explore meanings and values

acronym social GGRRAAAACCEEESSS, mentioned earlier, aims to assist practitioners in remaining mindful of all areas of difference. Burnham suggests that all these interrelated aspects of our identities and experience are important in influencing our experience of supervision, training, and practice. They also influence training contexts and the inherent power relationships between supervisors and supervisees. Hence it is useful to consider these aspects of diversity in the three levels of supervisory practice mentioned earlier: the general culture of supervision, the culture of the SR, and the culture of practice. Burnham, Alvis Palma, & Whitehouse (2008) suggest some helpful questions with which to approach exploring culture within the SR, for example:

- What similarities or differences are visible and voiced or invisible and unvoiced?
- Which social GRRAACCEEESSS are named or silenced?
- Which differences is it helpful to keep or integrate?

Burnham et al. (2008) conclude that social differences influence learning and that learning reciprocally influences difference. Learning is a process of questioning assumptions, reflecting, and challenging. This fundamental process of sharing, exploring, and checking assumptions within an SR suggests a form of collaboration that allows for the exploration of power. In a formal training context this can be seen as a way of achieving collaboration within traditional hierarchical relationships.

Summary and Conclusions

In this chapter we have discussed values-based practice, ethics, and cultural competence, and explored the links between them. We have covered a range of frameworks, models, and research to help us understand the multiple influences on the SR, and the role the SR has to play in effectively managing the complexity of this area. We have found the concept of "cultural humility" (Tervalon & Murray-Garcia, 1998) helpful in providing an overarching framework in approaching this discussion. This commitment to self-reflection and critique is essential to an ethical and diversity sensitive approach and links very closely to reflective practice, which is discussed in detail in Chapter 9. Cultural humility offers an approach to managing power and difference that is respectful and supports the supervisee in sharing their particular background and experience with the supervisor without being required to take on an expert role. Clearly this is facilitated by, and in turn facilitates, a strong open and respectful SR.

Key Points

- Values-based practice is important to developing good supervisory relationships; it encompasses a sensitivity and openness to the unique values and perspectives of both supervisor and supervisee.
- An ethical stance is also fundamental to effective supervisory relationships, and it is important that supervisors model ethically sensitive practice.
- Power is inherent in the supervisory relationship and should be negotiated.
- Common ethical dilemmas for supervisory relationships relate to confidentiality, boundaries, multiple relationships, competence, informed consent, due process, and multicultural competence
- The supervisory relationship can become a context in which to explore values and to consider ethical codes when considering dilemmas in practice.
- Cultural humility is important in supervisory relationships and involves a curiosity and openness to exploring cultural contexts sensitively and respectfully.

Part II

Effective Supervisory Relationships

Best Practice

6

Good Beginnings

The aims of this chapter are:

- to describe how to begin supervisory relationships well;
- to summarize how to develop a supervision contract that attends to the supervisory relationship.

We have learned over the years and the many supervisory relationships that we have supported in our professional roles, that starting well can prevent all sorts of relational strains. It is therefore essential for effective SRs that both parties prepare well and invest both professionally and emotionally in each new relationship. This provides the opportunity to apply some of the theory and evidence discussed in Part I to day-to-day practice. In this chapter, we focus on how to ensure a good beginning to the SR, and the central role of effective contracting in this process. An example of a supervision contract is included at the end of this chapter, which illustrates how to contract for the relationship in supervision.

Getting Things Off to a Good Start

Both supervisor and supervisee have a great deal to contribute to ensure that the SR begins well. Many of the characteristics that both parties bring to supervision have been summarized earlier (see Table 3.2 and Table 3.3). The supervisor can demonstrate a genuine interest in providing supervision and supporting the supervisee's learning and development, as well as a sensitivity to the challenges and stresses involved in the work. This communicates an important message to the supervisee—that supervision and the supervisee are important and valued. Similarly, a willingness to be known by the supervisee and an appropriate use of self-disclosure can help to promote collaboration in the SR and to manage power effectively.

If the supervisee is in training and the supervisor is providing a training placement, then some preparation ahead of the supervisee's arrival—in terms of planning induction activities to enable the supervisee to become acquainted

Effective Supervisory Relationships: Best Evidence and Practice, First Edition.
Helen Beinart and Sue Clohessy.

with the service setting, setting up learning opportunities, and spending time with the supervisee (Clohessy, 2008)—can also help to ensure that supervision and the SR begin well. In any team or wider organizational context, it is helpful to prepare the team for a new trainee or member of staff (regardless of experience). This can include practicalities such as arranging access to the essentials of the job (e.g., clients, desk, phone, computer) and alerting the team to role expectations and accountabilities. If external supervision is being provided (i.e., the supervisor is providing supervision to a supervisee who is not working in their setting), it is extremely helpful to explore mutual expectations so that the supervisor can gain an understanding of the organizational or other context in which the work is taking place, and the supervisor can explain their own background and working practices.

There are also many things that supervisees can also do to enable the SR to begin well. These include showing enthusiasm and an openness to learn, a willingness to reflect on their prior experiences, their learning needs, and how the supervisor can best support them (e.g., Clohessy, 2008). Supervisees may need to spend some time thinking about these issues in preparation for supervision. Supervisees may not always be aware of their learning needs or may not know what to expect, particularly if they have received little previous supervision. They may benefit from some preparatory reading about the service or practice area or about supervision itself. The exercise in Box 6.1 can be used to prepare for new SRs. Supervisees can be invited to do this and to share their learning in early contracting discussions with their supervisor.

Of course, it is also helpful for supervisors to prepare for a new SR, and we include an exercise later in this chapter to enable supervisors to reflect on their expectations, constraints, and values as they relate to the SR. Preparing for

---

Box 6.1 Questions to encourage supervisee preparation for a new supervisory relationship

- What has been your experience of supervision so far (duration, contexts, etc.)?

- Describe the supervisory relationships that have worked best for you in the past.

- What did these supervisors do that you valued?

- What are you hoping for from this supervisory relationship?

- Is there anything you are apprehensive about?

supervision and beginning the SR in this way communicate an important meta-message about the relationship. It demonstrates to supervisees that a supervisor is interested in and committed to their learning and development and to making the supervision work well; and to supervisors that a supervisee values what they have to offer, is enthusiastic and interested in learning, and is willing to be an active and collaborative partner in the SR. Indeed, there is some limited evidence that making a good start leads to the SR improving, or at least remaining homeostatic over time (Ladany, Walker, Pate-Carolan, & Evans, 2008).

Developing a Meaningful Supervision Contract

One of the most important ways to ensure that a SR starts well and continues to work effectively is to establish a meaningful supervision contract, which makes clear the mutual expectations of both supervisor and supervisee and other interested parties in the relationship (e.g., training institutions, professional bodies, working contexts).

According to Scaife (2009), the contracting process involves the supervisor and the supervisee reaching an agreement about the requirements of their working contexts, the timing and frequency of their contacts with each other, their role relationships and the purpose and process of supervision. Scaife suggests that it is important that contracting be seen as a dynamic, ongoing process, beginning at the point of establishing a supervisory relationship and open to renegotiation throughout its duration. For the contract to be meaningful it must be regularly reviewed. There may be a drive to rush this process, to develop a superficial contract quickly (or omit it completely), and to progress with discussing the supervisee's work in the supervision session. However, we would suggest that it is well worth investing time in the contracting process, particularly at the beginning of the SR. Doing so encourages supervisees to reflect on what they need from supervision, clarifies mutual expectations, and facilitates consideration about how this particular supervisory relationship will work. Supervisors can inform supervisees that much of the initial supervision session will be spent on contracting, or negotiate that contracting will form part of the agenda of the first couple of sessions, in addition to any work they are keen to bring to the supervision. It is helpful, early on in the SR, to explain the benefits of contracting and to provide a rationale for spending time on establishing a meaningful agreement on how you plan to work together.

Bernard and Goodyear (2014) suggest that contracting in supervision helps to orient and educate the supervisee about the different aspects of the SR, including informed consent (see Chapter 5). It can be a particularly useful document to refer back to if there is conflict or disagreement. Spending time on contracting can also encourage collaboration and openness between supervisor and supervisee (e.g., Osborn & Davies, 1996; Scaife, 2009).

Guidelines for developing supervision contracts often focus on pragmatic considerations (when and where supervision will take place, as well as the frequency and duration of the meetings), competence development, and the requirements of professional bodies (e.g., Gonsalvez, 2014) or ethical considerations (e.g., Thomas, 2007). Indeed, supervision contracts can help to articulate the roles and responsibilities of both supervisor and supervisee, and can help support ethical behavior through referencing relevant ethical guidelines (Osborn & Davies, 1996). There can be differing emphases in supervision contracts that range between agency structure, emphasizing compliance to agency rules (Munson, 2012), and developmental learning goals focused on meeting the needs of the supervisee (Osborn & Davis, 1996). These are all important issues to consider in the development of a contract between supervisor and supervisee, but the emphasis of this chapter will be on how to develop a contract that ensures a good start to the relationship, and sets a context in which the working relationship between supervisor and supervisee can be discussed, reviewed, and negotiated. We tend to refer to the development of a meaningful psychological contract for the SR alongside the more formal and practical agreements usually included in contracting.

What to Include in a Supervision Contract

The following is not intended as an exhaustive list but are suggestions of areas to consider when negotiating a contract with a supervisee. You are invited to add areas which will be important to cover in your own working contexts.

Pragmatics and Practicalities

Timing
Where, when, for how long, and how often will you meet? It is important to clarify frequency, duration, and any time boundaries that may impact the experience of the SR. It is particularly useful to discuss how you may manage missed or interrupted sessions. If either party is late for supervision, how will this be managed?

Personal Issues
What are the arrangements for contact outside of supervision if this is needed? What should supervisees do if urgent issues arise that cannot wait until the next supervision meeting? It is helpful to consider if, as a supervisor, you are willing to be contacted in an emergency and, if so, you should provide appropriate contact details. It is always useful to provide a contingency plan or back-up arrangements if the main supervisor is not available.

Contextual Issues
This may include issues specific to the context of your work, for example working hours, record-keeping, presentational issues such as dress code, and agency rules and practices. If there are issues particular to your working context, it is essential to communicate these to your supervisee at an early stage to ensure a good beginning.

These are some of the pragmatic issues to consider when setting up supervision. They are also some of the easiest to discuss because they are fairly uncontentious.

However, it is important that they are clear and understood because they form part of the boundaries of supervision, and help to facilitate the SR as a reliable and safe space within which the supervisee can reflect on their work.

Purpose of Supervision, Roles, and Responsibilities

A discussion of mutual expectations and the roles and responsibilities in the SR can be helpful. This provides an opportunity for the supervisor to share their understanding of the purposes and aims of supervision and the role of the supervisor. It is particularly important if supervisor and supervisee come from different professional backgrounds and may therefore also have different expectations about supervision. Depending on the context in which the SR is taking place, issues of clinical, professional, or management responsibility should also be clarified. If the supervisor has a formal evaluative role (if the supervisee is in training, for example), the requirements of the training institution should be discussed, as well as the expectations of the service or agency context. Clarifying what the supervisor expects from the supervisee is also a fruitful discussion, for example openness and honesty about their learning needs, preparation for supervision, as well as negotiating who will do what in supervision (e.g., who will keep notes). A full discussion on expectations is a useful way of establishing a set of goals and parameters for the SR.

As well as discussing roles and responsibilities, it is helpful to provide some background information about the supervisor, their style of work, experience, and preferred approaches to practice. In the United States, it is becoming more common for supervisors to provide a professional disclosure statement which may, for example, cover their qualifications and registrations, areas of professional competence, experience of training in and provision of supervision, and preferred models and methods of evaluation (Bernard & Goodyear, 2014).

Supervision Structure

It is helpful to discuss the expected structure of a supervision session. For example, many supervisors use an agenda to structure a session and expect a supervisee to think about and to prepare material prior to the session. Some supervisors expect a supervisee to bring a prepared supervision question to help focus the session so that they can make the best use of the time available. Often supervision agendas are developed collaboratively and supervisees need to be prepared for this. Some supervisors will begin by reflecting on issues from previous sessions, and will follow up on any agreed actions. It is helpful that this is communicated in advance to supervisees so that they can prepare accordingly. Many supervisory dyads also like to spend some time reflecting on the process of supervision itself, and this needs to be included in the agenda so that sufficient time is allowed for a meaningful discussion.

Goals and Evaluation or Monitoring

In training or professional registration contexts, competencies required will be established by the learning institution but, during contracting, these will need to be translated to individualized goals for the supervisee. It is also important to be clear about formative and summative methods of evaluation and any means that will be used. For example, direct observation, recordings, and specific measures are common ways of monitoring practice (see Chapter 7 for a full discussion of feedback and evaluation). The significant issue for the SR is that, regardless of the level of experience of the supervisee, it is important to be transparent about methods of evaluation and monitoring, including communication about how information may be shared.

Supervision has an important educational function, so identifying learning needs and competencies to be developed is an important part of the supervision contract. Supervisors and supervisees should both be aware of the competencies inherent in their professional role and supervisees should be encouraged to identify their associated goals for supervision. There is some suggestion that supervisees may set goals that are too general, and so supervisors should facilitate goal-setting (Gonsalvez, 2014). Gonsalvez also suggests that the asking of the questions, rather than how accurate the answers are, is most important because it facilitates self-awareness and reflective practice. Some questions that may facilitate this process are presented in Box 6.2.

In addition to specifying learning styles, competencies, and related goals, it can be useful to consider the learning methods that can be used in supervision. For example, experiential methods such as role play, the use of live observation, or observation by video or audio recordings, as well as case discussion and reflective questioning, are all methods that can be used in supervision to facilitate learning.

Box 6.2 Questions to help supervisees reflect on their learning needs

- What are your strengths? What are you good at?

- What would others say your strengths were? What would they notice about you?

- What are the areas you need to develop? What competencies do these relate to?

- What feedback have you been given in past supervision about areas you could focus on developing further?

- What learning opportunities would help you to develop these competencies?

Feedback

Feedback is such a core part of the learning process in supervision that it is crucial to begin to have discussions about feedback during the contracting phase of the SR. We have discussed the giving and receiving of effective feedback in detail in Chapter 7, and stress the importance of addressing experiences and expectations regarding feedback when contracting for the SR. Supervisees may be invited to reflect on their feedback preferences and on the types of feedback that help them develop or, conversely, lead to defensiveness. Supervisors can then tailor their feedback accordingly.

Similarly, establishing with the supervisee that you, as a supervisor, welcome feedback on supervision is also beneficial, even though giving feedback to supervisors can be much more challenging for supervisees because of issues of power. However, demonstrating an interest in the supervisee's perspective on what is working well and what could be done differently in supervision, models openness to feedback. In our experience, beginning discussions about feedback early on in SRs contributes to a collaborative working alliance.

Diversity

It is common practice in some modalities of supervision (e.g., systemic) to share cultural genograms in the early phase of supervision. Our discussion in Chapter 5 explores these issues in some depth. It is our experience that it is best to begin to broach differences in values and approaches as part of initial discussions if they are to be considered throughout the SR (see Chapter 9 for some examples of how to include discussions of diversity within the supervision contract).

Ethical Considerations

There are a number of ethical issues to consider in the supervision contract. A more comprehensive discussion of the ethical issues in supervision generally can be found in Chapter 5. Reference to ethical and professional guidelines and codes of conduct can be helpful in the contract, as can an acknowledgment that supervision is a safe place to explore ethical issues and to facilitate ethical decision-making skills.

Informed consent is as relevant to the supervisory relationship as it is to the therapeutic relationship in clinical contexts (Thomas, 2007), and there is some suggestion that it can improve the effectiveness and satisfaction of both supervisor and supervisee if the subject is addressed appropriately (e.g., Guest & Dooley, 1999). Being clear about the limits of confidentiality in supervision is important. What will be kept confidential, and what might need to be shared, are important to discuss, particularly if the SR is a training relationship and the supervisor has gate-keeping responsibilities and needs to make decisions about the supervisees' competence. Supervision can have competing demands at its core: supervisees are expected to be open about their dilemmas, learning needs, and mistakes, while supervisors have to create a safe space for them to do this, while also retaining their gate-keeping and evaluative roles. Discussion of confidentiality when contracting can facilitate this process and ensure that supervisors gain informed consent from their supervisees.

Learning Needs and Preferences

Exploring the supervisee's preferences for learning is also a helpful area to explore. According to learning theory (Kolb, 1984), we all have learning preferences (see Chapter 2 for more information about adult learning). Some may have a preference for learning through concrete experience (here-and-now activities such as role play), or reflective observation (an opportunity to plan and to reflect on experience before taking action). Others may have a preference for active conceptualization (understanding relevant theory and models) or active experimentation (learning through modeling and trying things out with detailed feedback). Supervisors may also have preferred learning styles, some of which may not always match well with those of their supervisees.

The Supervisory Relationship and Relational Considerations

Discussing how to make the supervisory relationship work well is perhaps the most fundamental part of contracting, given how important the SR is to effective supervision. Encouraging the supervisee to reflect on their past experiences of supervision, and specifically what they have found more and less helpful, can be useful. It can also be beneficial for supervisors to share some of their values and preferences with the supervisee, which requires some prior reflection on their own supervision experiences and their preferred supervision style. The questions in Box 6.3 may help supervisors to reflect on their supervision values, and can serve as good preparation for supervision.

These questions can help a supervisor prepare for supervision, either as a self-reflective exercise, or as a discussion in the supervisor's own supervision. It may not be necessary to use these questions to reflect before the beginning of every supervisory relationship, but a consideration of how a new supervisee may experience you as a supervisor, the similarities and differences between you both that may influence the SR, the impact of your work setting on you and the SR, and any feedback you have received on your supervision will be worth considering regularly.

Encouraging the supervisee to consider aspects of their background which may influence their work and the SR is also helpful, but it is also important that supervisees have control over what they disclose about themselves. Supervisees can be invited to share background information about themselves that they consider will be useful for the supervisor to know. Because of the hierarchical nature of the SR, it is worthwhile putting power on the agenda and providing opportunities to discuss how power can be used effectively to empower the supervisee and to support their learning. It is also useful to flag the possible misuse of power. On a related issue, it is also important to establish what will happen if there are difficulties in the SR, creating a context in which both supervisor and supervisee can review how the SR is developing and raise any issues as they arise (see Chapter 8).

Box 6.3 Questions to help supervisors reflect on their values and preferences

- What do I think is important in making supervision work well?

- What is my preferred theoretical orientation? How will this influence my supervision?

- Who are the supervisors who have most influenced my practice? Which of their qualities and characteristics would I like to hold onto?

- Have I had experiences of SRs with supervisors which have been more difficult? Which of these characteristics would I like to let go of in my own practice as a supervisor?

- What characteristics do I value in supervisees, e.g., openness, willingness to work hard?

- What am I likely to find more challenging?

- How might I come across to supervisees? Have I been given any feedback about supervision before?

- Are there similarities and differences between my supervisee and me that may influence supervision, e.g., age, gender, ethnicity?

- Are there issues or stressors in my work setting that are influencing me? How might they influence supervision and my relationship with my supervisee?

The questions in Box 6.4 are intended as a guide to help the development of the supervision contract with a focus on establishing the relationship. It may help give supervisees the opportunity to reflect on some of these issues as part of the contract and to return to them. As described earlier, there should also be discussions about the practicalities of supervision, roles and responsibilities, ethical considerations, and learning needs. It may be useful to allow supervisees to have some time to reflect on these issues. Once again, it is the process of asking

---

Box 6.4 Questions to help develop a contract for the supervisory relationship

- What background information would you like to share about yourself? What do you think it would be helpful for me to know about you?

- What have you valued about supervision in the past? What have your past supervisors done that you have appreciated or that has been helpful?

- Has there been anything you have found unhelpful about past supervision or anything your past supervisors did that was problematic for you?

- What do I value from supervisees?

- How do you prefer to be given feedback? What is the best way to give you feedback? How would you like me to tell you if there are areas I think you could improve on?

- How will I know if, for example, you are finding things difficult or if supervision is not meeting your needs?

- You might find me, for example, preoccupied or over-committed. If this impacts on our supervision, this is what you can do about it …

- How shall we remain mindful of issues of difference and diversity in our supervision, both in your work and in our work together?

- How can we address differences of opinion in supervision, or problems in our work together?

- How and when shall we review supervision?

---

questions and having the discussion that is perhaps more important than the accuracy of the answers. It communicates an important message from the supervisor to the supervisee, that supervision is an important, valued space and that their relationship is something to be negotiated and reviewed.

Reviewing the Contract

Once there have been some discussions about how supervision and the supervisory relationship will work, it is important to regularly check in, to review the contract, and to renegotiate if necessary. When and how frequently this should be done will depend on the nature of the SR, the parties involved, and the context within which the SR occurs. For example, a training SR may already have a particular structure because of the duration of the training placement or the expectations of the training course, so it may make sense to review the contract at intervals with this in mind. Supervisory relationships with qualified professionals may be more open-ended, so it can be helpful to discuss when the contract should be reviewed. Regular, informal checking in to see how supervision and the SR are working is important, but there should also be time scheduled for a more formal review of the SR to provide some time to reflect on the supervision process and to provide a forum for discussion of any issues that may arise. Again, reviewing the contract communicates the message that the SR is collaborative and can be negotiated, and that supervisors are invested in making it work well. Box 6.5 summarizes some questions that may help in reviewing the supervision contract.

Box 6.5 Reviewing the contract

- What has been working well in supervision?

- What has not been working so well?

- Is there anything we could be doing more or less of? Is there anything we could do differently?

- How has feedback been given and received? Has there been enough feedback?

- What progress has been made towards the original goals and/or learning needs we identified? Have they been met? What new goals or learning needs can we focus on next?

- What learning methods have we used? Have these been helpful? Should we try different methods?

- Is there anything about our SR that has been challenging? Is there anything we can discuss or address?

- What changes might we need to make to our supervision contract, in light of the above?

The following is an example of a first supervision session with a new trainee psychologist (Maya) that illustrates some of the issues described in this chapter, followed by an opportunity to reflect on the conversation (Box 6.6). An example of a supervision contract developed between Maya and her supervisor (Ana) is included at the end of this chapter.

SUPERVISOR:	I would like to start by spending some time getting to know one another and exploring expectations about how we may work together.
SUPERVISEE:	Umm, OK … I'm not really quite sure what to expect …
SUPERVISOR:	Perhaps it would help if I told you a little bit about my working context and myself.
SUPERVISEE:	Yes, that would be great, thanks …
SUPERVISOR:	Well, I've worked with children and young people for 10 years and this is my second job. I have been working in this area for a couple of years. I am passionate about making psychological services available to as many young people as possible, normalizing distress so it's no more difficult to seek psychological help than seeing a GP. That's been quite a challenge given the resources available and I sometimes get really frustrated. I am really pleased that you have come to work with us because I like supervising and we appreciate an extra pair of hands.
SUPERVISEE:	(intake of breath) I have no experience working with children so I am not sure how much use I will be to you. Actually, I have very little experience of children all together and find them a little scary.
SUPERVISOR:	That's OK. I don't expect you to run before you can walk and it's really helpful for me to know that you are a feeling a little anxious—how can I support you with this?
SUPERVISEE:	I don't know really. I'm a bit worried about being thrown in the deep end.
SUPERVISOR:	Don't worry—lots of trainees find kids a bit scary. Perhaps you would like to shadow me for the first couple of weeks? It will give us a chance to get to know each other. We could also set up opportunities for you to visit clinics or schools and meet other staff. There are quite a few newer members of the team and I am sure you will be able to support one another …
SUPERVISEE:	That sounds great but I don't want to be a burden to you, particularly as you are so busy.
SUPERVISOR:	Well, let's do a deal; it's really important to me that you keep me briefed about how you are getting on. I want to be able to trust that you can be honest with me—I feel you have made a really good start. I enjoy supervising and I

hope by the time you leave you will be as passionate about the work as I am ... what would be burdensome to me is if I felt you were not being open with me. Perhaps you could tell me a little about your experience and what you have found helpful in supervision in the past ...

SUPERVISEE: I have been working with adults with mental health problems for the past year—I absolutely loved it—particularly the more complex cases. I like the challenge of the work and the privilege of hearing people's stories. I worked with one young mother who had experienced a severe trauma just after she had her second child. I was quite anxious about exploring this to start off with, but my previous supervisor gently encouraged me and helped me develop strategies to approach the issues ...

SUPERVISOR: So, it sounds like you have quite a lot of experience working with complexity in families—very similar to the work here—you may surprise yourself. It also sounds like you thrive on a balance of support and challenge, which I hope we will be able to provide for you but it will be up to you to help me get this balance right so it meets your needs ...

Box 6.6 Reflections on vignette

- Note down how the supervisor began to establish rapport. What methods were used?

The supervisor initiated the conversation by sharing information about their work values, expectations, and frustrations. She was able to demonstrate a genuine enthusiasm both for the work and for supervision. This may have been a bit daunting for the supervisee but it allowed the disclosure of anxieties about the client group and worry about being a burden. This, in turn, gave the supervisor the opportunity to normalize her anxieties and ask how she could best support the supervisee. The supervisor was able to flag her expectation of honesty within the SR and to praise the supervisee for starting well. They were also able to begin to address supervisee learning needs and preferences for feedback, as well as to establish the supervisor's expectation that the supervisee did not need to be expert in the work but did need to take responsibility for collaborating and giving feedback within the SR. The message was encouraging but also set a series of expectations.

This early session demonstrates several of the key aspects of establishing the SR—spending time, listening and attending, containment, openness, investment and encouragement, beginning to share values and expectations, setting a sense of a collaborative endeavor which has an overarching purpose of providing a service as well as supporting supervisee learning.

Conclusion

The development of an agreement about mutual expectations and working practices through contracting is, in our view, the most important way of establishing an effective SR. In this chapter we have reviewed the significance of contracting for the SR and have provided some guidance about the areas that may be covered. We have also provided some useful practical guidance and examples of questions that may facilitate these discussions. We have stressed throughout this chapter that contracting should be understood as an initial agreement and as an ongoing review process within the SR rather than as a formal document. In many ways, we see it as setting the agenda for the SR by raising potential issues that can be explored more fully as the relationship develops. It is the process of the discussions, the openness and curiosity, the interest and commitment that set the tone for a truly collaborative SR, and ensure good beginnings.

Example of a Supervision Contract for the SR

The following is an example of a beginning supervision contract between a trainee psychologist (Maya) and her supervisor (Ana). This example emphasizes the relational aspects of supervision.

The aims of supervision are:

- to provide support and challenge for Maya's learning in a safe relationship;
- to focus on building Maya's competencies and confidence in working with children and families;
- for Maya to meet the competency requirements of the training course for working with children, young people and their families, and to adhere to the working policies and practices of the Child and Family Centre as discussed in supervision.

Contexts

Child and Family Centre: Maya will be on placement Wednesdays–Fridays, 9a.m.–5p.m. Annual leave and study leave from placement to be discussed in advance. Maya to familiarize herself with working policies of the clinic (e.g., record-keeping, confidentiality, safeguarding, lone worker policy, etc.) and to abide by these. Ana to provide these policies and any support Maya might need.

An induction program will be arranged for Maya to meet the team and familiarize herself with the team culture

Training institution: Maya to carry her own caseload of individual children and families, with a variety of presenting problems. There are also opportunities for teamwork, working with a parent support group, teaching, research and audit, and service development. An audit of group work is much needed and Maya is interested in developing this as she has previous experience in service audit.

An appropriate range and amount of work will be provided, and Ana will provide regular weekly supervision of at least an hour. Maya will keep a record of her clinical activity on placement, and will also write up a case for academic submission. Ana will read a draft of this and provide feedback. A tutor from the training institution will visit twice throughout the course of the placement to review Maya's progress, and to monitor the quality of the training placement.

Learning Needs and Interests

Maya has little prior experience of working with children and their families, and is looking for some general experience in the area, and an opportunity to build her confidence. She has experience of working with adults in mental health outpatient settings, and is interested in working with psychological trauma. She would like to explore this interest in children and families.

Learning preferences: Maya and Ana will use the Learning Styles Inventory to explore learning preferences. Maya prefers not to be "thrown in at the deep end," and likes an opportunity to observe first. They agree to build on existing strengths and to work toward developing new learning and challenge.

Roles, Responsibilities, and Values

Ana is an experienced supervisor and has been trained in supervision by the Training Institute. She enjoys supervising, and is keen to give Maya a positive experience in her field. Ana will provide regular weekly supervision, and is willing to be contacted outside of formal supervision times if Maya needs additional support. Additionally, back-up cover will be arranged with a senior member of the team. She will book a room for their supervision, and will collaboratively set an agenda with Maya at the beginning of each meeting and keep her own supervision records, including a list of agreed actions. She has an evaluative role in supervision, and will provide regular feedback about any areas that she thinks Maya needs to develop. They will collaboratively develop specific goals as learning needs become apparent. She will support Maya to develop the required competencies. She values openness and honesty and will appreciate Maya being open about her uncertainties and her mistakes.

Maya has had positive experiences of supervision during her training. She likes an opportunity to observe her supervisors initially, before she takes on work independently. She is nervous about working with children, as this is a new area for her. She will prepare for supervision by spending time in advance thinking about what she needs from Ana, for example questions she has about her work, and will use this to inform her agenda-setting with Ana at the beginning of supervision. She will keep her own supervision records, including a list of agreed actions from her discussions with Ana.

Goals and Learning Methods

General goals will follow the competency requirements of the training institution. Specific goals will be specified later in the contract.

Mutual observation and joint working at the beginning of the training placement will provide opportunities for getting to know each other and our ways of working.

Opportunities for live observation and use of tape recordings of Maya's work are expected throughout the training placement.

Feedback

Feedback preferences: Maya prefers a combination of direct feedback on her learning needs, and would like some help noticing her strengths, as she has a tendency to be self-critical. Ana values feedback on her supervision, and will ask for this regularly. They will review how feedback is given and received at regular intervals.

Formal evaluation will be in line with the competency requirements and evaluation methods of the training institution.

Consideration of Difference and Diversity

Ana and Maya will make time in supervision to consider the similarities and differences in their cultural backgrounds, and how this may influence their work. They will share their cultural genograms in supervision to facilitate reflective practice, and keep in mind social GRRAACCCEEESSS throughout Maya's placement—both in Maya's work with service users, and in their work together in supervision.

Ethical Considerations

Both Maya and Ana will abide by the code of ethics and conduct specified by the British Psychological Society. Supervision will be a safe context in which they can explore the ethical issues in Maya's clinical work, and consider ethical decision-making.

What is discussed in supervision will remain confidential, with some provisos. Ana will be required to formally evaluate Maya's progress, and so a summary of this learning and associated evidence (which may come from discussions in supervision) will be provided to the training institution. Additionally, if any issues are raised that cause significant concern (either for Ana or for Maya), for example professional practice issues, these may also be shared with the training institution. This will be discussed in supervision in advance. Ana may also discuss her supervision of Maya with her own supervisor, to ensure that she is providing the most helpful supervision

Managing Difficulties in Supervision

Both Ana and Maya are committed to making their supervisory relationship work well. They will review supervision every month to ensure that it is working effectively, and reflect on any problems which may arise. Any difficulties in the supervisory relationship will be approached with openness and curiosity, and seen as an opportunity for mutual learning. If they are unable to resolve any problems in the SR themselves, they will consider inviting a third party (such as a tutor from the Training Institution) to facilitate further discussions.

Pragmatics

Supervision will take place on Fridays 9:30 a.m.–10:30 a.m. at the Child and Family Centre. Ana is willing to be contacted outside of this time if Maya needs additional support. If Ana is on holiday, or off sick, she will arrange for supervision to be provided by another member of the Psychology Team.

Signed: ....

....

Key Points

- Preparing in advance for a new supervisory relationship is helpful for both supervisors and supervisees.
- Investing in the relationship, particularly at the beginning, is key.
- Contracting is a fundamental process in establishing and maintaining supervisory relationships, and it is important to spend time on this at the beginning of the relationship and to review it regularly.
- Contracting provides an opportunity to demonstrate how to have an open and collaborative conversation about the relationship.
- In addition to the practicalities of supervision, contracting should include a discussion of relevant background and cultural information about supervisor and supervisee, mutual expectations, learning needs and preferences for feedback, how to make the supervisory relationship work well, and how to address problems if they arise.

7

Giving and Receiving Feedback

The aims of this chapter are:

- to summarize research and best practice in giving and receiving feedback;
- to describe different methods of feedback;
- to discuss the role of the supervisory relationship in giving and receiving feedback.

In detailed studies of what supervisors actually do in supervision, feedback has been found to be the most common method used (Milne, 2009). In systematic reviews of supervision, 81% of supervisors reported using feedback methods such as praise and constructive criticism. Feedback is so central to supervision that several authors incorporate it within their definitions; for example, Milne (2007) refers to "corrective feedback," and Bernard and Goodyear (2014) to "evaluation." Many supervisors also report that they find feedback the most challenging aspect of supervision, probably because it is so central to the evaluative role. Indeed, supervisees often report that the quality and quantity of feedback received influences their experience of the supervisory relationship (Bernard & Goodyear, 2014). Specifically, balanced, clear, and direct feedback can increase satisfaction with supervision (Lehrman-Waterman & Ladany, 2001).

Hoffman, Hill, Holmes, and Freitas (2005, p. 3) define feedback in supervision as "information that supervisors give supervisees about their skills, attitudes, behavior and appearance that may influence their performance with clients or affect the SR." Feedback can be direct (e.g., "I noticed that you did not appear very confident at that point") or indirect (e.g., "I wonder how confident you were feeling at that point"). Similarly, Scaife (2009, p. 318) defines feedback as "a response or reaction providing useful information or guidelines for further action and development." Both these definitions regard feedback as central to professional learning and development. We would also add that, within the SR, feedback that supervisees give their supervisors is key, and mutual feedback is at the heart of truly collaborative and effective SRs. Creating a safe space in which supervisees feel empowered to give feedback to their supervisors is an important task in the SR.

Many theories of psychological change acknowledge the key role of feedback in learning and development. For example, in learning theory feedback is proposed to increase the frequency of the behavior it follows; and in systems

Effective Supervisory Relationships: Best Evidence and Practice, First Edition.
Helen Beinart and Sue Clohessy.
© 2017 John Wiley & Sons Ltd. Published 2017 by John Wiley & Sons Ltd.

theory feedback is the central mechanism of change. Feedback is a central part of effective supervision and it is crucial to learn how to do it as effectively as possible. It is widely accepted that feedback is most helpful in the context of a supportive and trusting relationship (Scaife, 2009).

Types of Feedback

There are several different types of feedback that are used within the SR including summative and formative feedback. Self-assessment, constructive challenge, and the use of self-report measures are also useful adjuncts to giving and receiving feedback.

Supervisors are likely to find summative or evaluative feedback—when they have to make a judgment of competence against a set of pre-defined criteria—most challenging. This is typical of the supervisory requirement for pre-qualification training or for those seeking professional registration or accreditation. This gate-keeping role can be uncomfortable, particularly if it involves feeding back on poor performance. We would also argue that monitoring and feedback supervisory responsibilities continue throughout a professional career. For example, highlighting poor practice or unethical behavior is an important function of supervision regardless of supervisee status (trainee or qualified). Formative feedback, defined as the process of facilitating skill acquisition and professional growth through feedback (Robiner, Fuhrman, & Ristvedt, 1993) is particularly significant for SRs. Formative feedback is focused on development and progress, whereas summative feedback focuses on outcomes.

Most texts on supervision include chapters on evaluation (e.g., Bernard & Goodyear, 2014) or assessment (e.g., Corrie & Lane, 2015; Scaife, 2009). However, we have chosen to focus in this chapter on learning the skills of giving and receiving effective feedback. Research by the Oxford Supervision Research Group (Beinart, 2002; see Chapter 2) explored how the evaluative role influenced SRs in a sample of trainee and recently qualified clinical psychologists. Interestingly, we found that, in those SRs rated as most effective, the role of evaluation was seen as normative. These participants had received regular formative feedback throughout and "knew where they stood," and consequently the summative element "contained no surprises." The opposite was true for the SRs rated as least effective. These supervisees reported feeling unsafe and experienced supervisors' evaluations as untrustworthy. Beinart (2002) found that the qualitative descriptors of receiving feedback in an unsafe SR were highly emotionally charged, and concluded that, where formative feedback is ongoing and is managed effectively within the SR, the evaluative role can be less daunting and more constructive for all concerned. Koh (2008) also emphasizes the importance of regular formative feedback and assessment for nurse education. In this chapter, we explore research and strategies for best practice in giving and receiving feedback, as well as providing some practical exercises and examples. We discuss the use of self-assessment, constructive challenge, and measures as adjuncts for effective feedback. Finally, we consider how to invite and encourage feedback from supervisees in order to work toward effective and collaborative SRs. The chapter ends with a summary of best practice in effective feedback.

Research Findings

Despite the centrality of feedback to the supervision process, there is remarkably little research specifically on feedback within supervision. Lehrman-Waterman and Ladany (2001) developed a measure of evaluation processes in supervision in which goal-setting and feedback were the two factors identified as important by their sample of supervisees. The limited research into supervisee preferences for feedback suggests that balanced, timely, objective, consistent, clear, and credible feedback in the context of a supportive relationship is experienced as most effective (Heckman-Stone, 2004). In general, supervisees report receiving too little feedback and this lack of feedback appears to affect the value they place on supervision (Lehrman-Waterman & Ladany, 2001).

Ladany and Melincoff (1999), in their study of non-disclosure in the SR, found that almost all (98%) of their sample of supervisors withheld feedback from their supervisees, most commonly concerning negative reactions to supervisees' professional performance or to their performance within supervision. Ladany and Melincoff suggest that supervisors do not give feedback for a number of reasons, such as preferring to avoid confrontation, concerns about the negative impact of feedback on the supervisee or on the SR, a belief that supervisees will discover the issues themselves when they are developmentally ready, and worries about the potential risk of turning supervision into therapy. The exercise in Box 7.1 provides an opportunity for the reader to reflect on feedback that they may have withheld, and the reasons for this.

In their qualitative study exploring supervisors' perspectives of feedback that was easy to give, difficult, or withheld, Hoffman et al. (2005) found that the majority of supervisors of doctoral counseling interns found it easier to give feedback about clinical issues. The content of feedback that was more difficult to give varied and included concerns about personal or professional behavior and problems within the SR. Supervisors had similar goals in providing feedback that were aimed at improving clinical practice, addressing personal or professional issues, or addressing a specific issue within the SR. Supervisors tended to use

---

Box 7.1 Reflective exercise on providing feedback

Think about a recent experience of giving feedback to a supervisee.

- What aspects of the feedback did you find easier or more difficult to provide?

- Was there anything you felt unable to provide feedback on?

- If so, what was the nature of the feedback you withheld?

direct feedback methods for the issues concerning clinical skills and *indirect* feedback methods for personal or professional issues and the SR. Feedback was withheld if the costs were felt to outweigh benefits, or if there were concerns about the quality of the SR. Facilitating conditions for providing feedback included the strength of the SR, supervisee openness, a clear need for feedback, timing, and supervisor sense of expertise or competence. Generally, when feedback was given, regardless of whether it was easy or difficult to give, outcomes were typically positive. However, when feedback was withheld outcomes were typically negative. In this study, supervisors clearly found it easier to give feedback to some supervisees than others and the quality of the SR seemed to be the significant factor. "It appeared that the supervision relationship that had developed between the two people was a major contributor to what made it easier to give feedback" (Hoffman et al., 2005, p. 11). These SRs were characterized by mutual shared goals, good rapport, valuing each other, and the supervisee's openness to feedback. It was suggested that the establishment of agreed goals facilitated greater openness (see Box 7.2 for an exercise on feedback and the quality of the SR).

The development of shared goals is also highlighted in the medical and nursing literature on feedback, where it is suggested that the learner and supervisor establish shared learning objectives, and that feedback should be based on these (Wood, 2000). Furthermore, Clynes and Raftery (2008) suggest that providing feedback to nursing students has a broader professional impact than improved clinical practice, including an increased sense of direction, confidence, motivation, and self-esteem. For supervisors, it is suggested that there are benefits too in providing feedback. These may include promoting professional growth and development, as well as enhanced interpersonal and communication skills. Both these studies stress the importance of training supervisors to provide effective feedback.

Box 7.2 Reflective exercise on giving feedback and the supervisory relationship

- Can you remember a SR where it was easy to give feedback regardless of the content?

- Can you describe the qualities of this SR?

- Did shared goals or expectations play a part?

- Were these goals individually tailored or externally set (e.g., a competency requirement?)

Hattie and Timperley (2007), in their seminal paper on the power of feedback in learning, argue that effective feedback must answer three major questions:

- Where am I going (goals)?
- How am I going (progress)?
- Where to next (actions)?

These questions relate to a number of different levels that include an understanding of how to perform a task (process level), a regulatory or meta-cognitive level, and the self or personal level. They argue that, for feedback to be effective, it has to be targeted at an appropriate level for the learner. However, they suggest that external feedback targeted at the personal level is rarely effective and that self-assessment is more effective at this level. Self-assessment (comprising self-appraisal and self-management) is a powerful self-regulatory mechanism for feedback. *Self-appraisal* reflects the learner's ability to review and evaluate their skills through self-monitoring. *Self-management* involves regulating behavior through planning, self-correction, and so on. These capacities are important as they guide the learner to know when to seek and receive feedback, and are likely to make them more receptive. However, there is a cost–benefit analysis in a learner seeking feedback. The benefit is in improving practice through reducing the gap between current and desired or expected performance. The costs may include effort, potential for shame or loss of face, and the risk of receiving poorly targeted or unhelpful feedback. When the cost–benefit ratio becomes prohibitive, people refrain from seeking feedback. However, effective feedback can enhance self-efficacy and lead to more effective self-regulation, so that the learner invests more effort and commitment to the task. Hattie and Timperley (2007) suggest that this rarely occurs when feedback is targeted at the person rather than at the task or process of learning. See Box 7.3 for a cost–benefit analysis on seeking feedback.

There is a small amount of research to suggest that feedback experiences may be culturally bound. For example, De Luque and Sommer (2000) found that learners from collectivist cultures preferred indirect and implicit feedback focused on the group rather than the self. Learners from individualist cultures preferred more direct, individual-focused feedback. However, Burkard, Knox, Clarke, Phelps, and Inman (2014) report that supervisors struggle to provide

---

Box 7.3 Exercise on the benefits and costs of seeking feedback

Think of a time when you avoided asking for feedback.

- Can you reflect on the cost–benefit ratio of this experience for you at the time?

- In retrospect, what, if anything, would you do differently?

direct feedback in cross-ethnic or interracial SRs and that supervisees welcome specific feedback and, where it was successfully provided, the SR was strengthened.

Methods to Support Effective Feedback

Contracting Goals and Feedback Preferences

The literature on feedback is clear about the importance of setting clear goals and identifying competencies to be developed. In some circumstances, such as during training or professional registration, the training or professional body will provide an externally agreed set of competencies that they require. However, to turn these into useful goals for your supervision, a conversation needs to take place during the contracting phase of the SR to establish mutually agreed objectives. The goals need to be personalized to fit with the learning needs and style of the supervisee. Ideally goals should be clearly worded and specific, and also achievable and feasible within the available capacity and resources. The dyad needs to agree the right balance between support and challenge to ensure that optimal learning takes place. As we have already discussed in the chapter on contracting (Chapter 6), continuous review and checking of the contract is helpful, and it is worthwhile to clarify specific goals or questions in each supervisory meeting.

However, there is another important task associated with feedback during contracting and this involves a discussion on feedback preferences. Feedback is easier to give if the supervisee is seen as open and receptive to it. Supervisees are more likely to be receptive if there have been some discussions about their preferences in being given feedback. This may relate to a discussion about learning styles (see Chapters 2 and 9). For example, a more reflective learner may prefer to have time to think through feedback and to discuss any issues after having had time to process and reflect. A more active learner may prefer a more active method such as trying things out here and now through role play or other methods. Some supervisees prefer their feedback to be direct and to the point, while others prefer a more gentle and tentative approach (see Box 7.4 for an exercise on feedback preferences). The important message here is that taking a meta-perspective about feedback allows for a discussion which recognizes and values different preferences, and encourages feedback about feedback, so that it can be adjusted if necessary. It can become a collaborative endeavor where the supervisee shares some of the responsibility for shaping the feedback to meet their learning needs at different points in their development. It is also worth considering the possibility of blind spots or defensiveness, so that even if feedback is delivered "expertly" according to a supervisee's preferences, it may still not be heard as intended.

It is our experience that supervisors and supervisees often get stuck in repeated patterns, such as the one described in the feedback vignette in Box 7.5, particularly in longer-term SRs. It can be quite helpful for a supervisor to note and reflect on these. This may not always be the easiest option and there may be some resistance on both sides—there is a certain comfort in repeating patterns

---

Box 7.4 Receiving helpful or less helpful feedback

Think about times when you have been given feedback.

- What characterized helpful feedback for you?

- What helped you "hear" the feedback, that is, take it on board?

- What characterized the feedback that was less helpful?

Box 7.5 Feedback vignette

A supervisee repeatedly requests feedback from a supervisor, seeking reassurance and asking if she could have done anything differently in managing a challenging client dynamic. The supervisor notes a feeling of exasperation and a sense of a repeating pattern of reassurance seeking and reassurance giving. It appears that, despite providing regular and specific feedback about what the supervisee had done well and possible alternative strategies to explore with the client, the supervisee does not appear to be hearing the feedback. The supervisor refers back to the contracting discussion on feedback where it was agreed that feedback would be reviewed regularly to check if it was meeting the supervisee's needs. She realizes that they have not reviewed the feedback and considers that it is time to do so. She tentatively raises the possibility of review with the supervisee, reminding her that they had agreed to "check out" regularly. The supervisee reports that there are no problems and that she values the feedback from the supervisor. The supervisor thanks the supervisee but wonders if the supervisee may be feeling a little stuck working with that particular group of people and if there is anything she can do differently to support her with this. The supervisee appears visibly relieved and they are able to have a discussion about how she is also feeling exasperated; they agree that a review with the client may be a useful avenue to explore. The supervisee acknowledges how helpful it has been to review the process of feedback as it allowed her to own her feelings of frustration and think about an alternative approach with her client.

---

even if they are not entirely helpful. In the vignette described in Box 7.5, the supervisor notes her sense of frustration and this prompts her to initiate a review. The supervisee initially appears defensive and attempts to evade feedback by praising the supervisor (see Box 7.6 for an exercise on feedback and defensiveness). The supervisor trusts her instincts and provides tentative feedback and an offer of support that allows progress to be made.

Box 7.6 Exercise on feedback and defensiveness

- Take some time to think about a piece of feedback that made you feel defensive.

- Describe what you noticed about your response, for example, were you hurt or angry?

- Was this a typical or an atypical response to feedback?

- Describe how that feedback was given.

- How could the other party have provided the feedback in a way that made you more receptive or open to learning?

Giving feedback to supervisees may be anxiety-provoking at times, particularly if you are unsure how it will be received. It can be helpful to clarify the feedback that you would like to give, and to practice this, perhaps in your own supervision or with a trusted colleague. The questions in Box 7.7 may help with this process.

We all have vulnerabilities about feedback and it is sometimes a question not just of providing it sensitively and skillfully, but also of making sure that it is well received. This requires the supervisee to be willing to comment on the impact of the feedback. In robust SRs it is quite possible to play with these ideas and to explore different methods and examples of feedback together. A good way of judging the strength of the SR is whether you feel you need to be careful before giving feedback or whether the relationship feels robust enough for you to get it a bit wrong and recover—often through humor or sharing narratives, or simply by checking in with one another. A supervisor who is able to model humility, and to show that it is acceptable to make mistakes and to learn from them, sends a powerful message to the supervisee about how they can use supervision. A strong SR is essential to support effective feedback.

Supervision Feedback Process and Structure

A method termed the "feedback sandwich" is a useful strategy in attempting to balance positive and negative feedback. The term was coined by Dohrenwend (2002) to describe how negative feedback can be sandwiched between two specific pieces of positive feedback. This method is thought to be particularly useful for novice supervisees or those with low confidence or self-esteem. However, Dohrenwend argues that in a strong SR this is not always needed.

Box 7.7 Questions to help prepare for giving feedback

- What specific information do you want to feed back? Can you provide examples?

- What behavior do you want to see changed?

- What do you think is the impact of this behavior—positive and negative?

- What would you prefer your supervisee to do differently?

- What learning goals would you like to set?

- What positive feedback would you like to offer?

A recent paper by James (2015) argues that the feedback sandwich is outdated and that a more effective approach is to engage the learner as an active partner in the learning process. He argues that negative feedback should generally be avoided in favor of constructive support and specific descriptive balanced feedback. New learning should be consolidated by practice or simulation. In general, feedback should be task- rather than person-focused, but if it is person-focused it should relate to effort rather than ability.

Wiggins (1998) describes the best feedback as highly specific and descriptive of what actually occurred, including examples from practice. Feedback should be clear and offered in terms of specific goals and standards. Feedback should focus on work performance and not on the recipient's character or personality. Similarly, Hawkins and Shohet (2012) use the mnemonic CORBS (clear, owned, regular, balanced, specific) to describe how supervision should be delivered. This is discussed in more detail later.

Many authors, particularly those from the field of education, describe discrete stages in the feedback process. For example, Jerome (1994) describes the following stages:

- providing a description of current behaviors that you want to reinforce and redirect to improve a situation;
- identifying specific situations where these behaviors have been observed;
- describing impacts and consequences of the current behaviors;
- identifying alternative behaviors and actions.

Pendleton, Schofield, Tate, and Havelock (1984) describe a collaborative feedback process whereby the learner is an active participant. They suggest seven steps in delivering feedback:

- The supervisor ensures that the learner is aware of the purpose of the feedback.
- The supervisor invites the learner to comment about their goals during their task.
- The learner shares what aspects of the task they think have been done well.
- The supervisor feeds back what aspects they think have been done well.
- The learner states what can be improved.
- The supervisor states what can be improved.
- The supervisor and learner agree action plans for improvement.

Similarly, the problem-based feedback process described by Vassilas and Ho (2000) includes the following steps:

- setting an agenda;
- ensuring the learner is aware of the function of the session;
- encouraging self-assessment and problem-solving;
- providing clear descriptive feedback;
- providing balanced feedback (what worked well and what could be done differently);
- suggesting alternatives, using modeling and rehearsal (e.g., role play);
- providing a clear summary of the learning points at the end.

All of these feedback processes have certain features in common including clarifying the purpose of the feedback; identifying strengths, needs, and possible actions, and (in the latter two models) inviting the learner's self-assessment before giving feedback. We shall now discuss self-assessment in a little more detail.

Self-assessment

The value of inviting self-assessment cannot be underestimated, as it provides the supervisor with a valuable insight into the supervisee's ability to evaluate their own performance, and identify their strengths and limitations (Clynes, 2004). If we apply Hattie and Timperley's (2007) model, described earlier, self-assessment is key to supervisee receptivity to feedback. Some authors argue that not all supervisees are able to accurately self-assess and have been found to either over- or underestimate their abilities, particularly if they are at an early developmental level in their professional development (Barnes, 2004). However, Sobell, Manor, Sobell, and Dum (2008) found that self-critique led to more openness to receiving supervisor feedback, and proposed this method to reduce defensiveness in the learner and to strengthen the SR. We have already established that, for feedback to be effective, the recipient needs to be open to receiving the feedback, and self-assessment may be one way of engaging the supervisee in this process, possibly through connecting with their issues or cognitive style. It could be argued that one of the key aspects of supervision is to support and develop the supervisee's capacity to self-assess as well as their ability to accurately appraise their own performance. There is much overlap here with reflective practice, which is discussed more fully in Chapter 9.

Constructive Challenge

Scaife (2009, p. 320) draws a helpful distinction between feedback and challenge, and sees challenge as "an invitation or undertaking to test one's capabilities to the full. Supervisors might thus challenge supervisees to use their identified strengths and capabilities, suggesting how these might be developed further." Scaife notes that novice supervisees may have difficulty identifying their own strengths, and a supervisor can help by describing the capabilities that they observe and encouraging the supervisee to apply these more widely and in different contexts. For example, a supervisor may identify a pre-determined competency and support the supervisee in self-assessing their performance, seeking evidence of progress thus far and further areas in which this competency could be applied. This approach, adapted from positive psychology, enables the supervisor to challenge strengths rather than weaknesses in order to foster the supervisee's learning and development. Scaife (2009) suggests that this method of feedback is less likely to trigger defensiveness but notes that it may not be an appropriate method if there are serious concerns about performance or conduct.

Scaife (2009) suggests some principles and steps to support effective challenging. These are summarized as follows:

- identify and keep in mind the purpose of the challenge—the desired learning outcome;
- establish a SR where there is mutual respect and which is based on supervisee learning needs;
- encourage self-challenge and show an openness to being challenged yourself;
- decide whether you have the authority to challenge (have you discussed and agreed this method of learning in your SR contract?);
- build on success, however small, and encourage the supervisee to notice and develop their strengths;
- get your facts clear—do some further information-gathering if necessary—and be specific in your feedback;
- practice making clear and direct statements—be authentic;
- consider starting sentences with "I"—this clarifies that it is your opinion; "you" statements are often received as criticisms or judgments;
- use immediacy to reflect on the process of the SR if needed (e.g., "My challenge was intended to help you develop *x* skill but it does not appear to be helping you, can we approach it from another angle that would be more helpful to you?");
- offer to come back to the issue after time to reflect;
- try role reversal to open up solutions if you are feeling stuck;
- be prepared to show humility and model a non-defensive approach—supervisors often get a little anxious about challenging and this can impact on how the feedback is delivered.

The use of challenge as a method of feedback is a helpful way to encourage supervisees to take a more active role in their learning and development, and creates opportunities for their learning to be stretched. It has the advantage of providing clear and realistic expectations, and, by focusing on strengths, it may be experienced as somewhat less judgmental and be less likely to trigger a defensive reaction.

In their discussion of delivering feedback to nursing students, Myrick and Yonge (2002) also stress the importance of building on strengths. They suggest that feedback should encourage students to become confident and competent in developing a plan that achieves safe and effective nursing care. They suggest approaching the student with sensitivity and taking on a helping rather than a corrective role. It is stressed that feedback should be given in private, when there is time and opportunity for clarification and discussion.

Conn (2002) makes the important point not to confuse feedback with praise. While praise may be conducive to developing a positive SR, it may not provide the supervisee with specific insights into their performance and how they may improve.

Encouraging Supervisee Feedback

Although supervisors may find feedback and evaluation challenging, it is generally more challenging for supervisees to give feedback to their supervisor. The SR has a power dynamic (partly influenced by the monitoring and evaluation function of the supervisor role) that has a significant impact on inhibiting open and honest feedback from the supervisee. The single most effective way of managing this is by developing a SR that is safe enough for the supervisee to be honest, and to trust that you, as a supervisor, will deal with any feedback in a constructive way. Many supervisees avoid giving honest feedback to their supervisors for fear of receiving negative evaluations. Creating a relational context in which feedback is welcomed and responded to is one way of encouraging supervisee feedback. This should be addressed early within the SR when developing the contract, so that permission for feedback to be given is clearly established and feedback is invited by the supervisor. It is helpful to share the expectation of mutual feedback and to begin to practice this throughout the SR by regularly checking in with one another. It may also be helpful to be aware of, and to raise, some of your own limitations (e.g., being over-committed) and to invite the supervisee to let you know if this has an impact on them. It is essential to be clear about the goals of supervision and how the evaluative elements will be conducted so that the supervisee knows what to expect and can collaborate in making this work well.

Our experience is that supervisees very rarely initiate feedback and it is generally down to the supervisor to ask for it. Some suggestions for questions that may aid this process are described in Box 7.8. We strongly encourage supervisory dyads to engage in conversations about their experience of feedback. Taking a meta-perspective provides an opportunity to reflect together on the process of giving and receiving feedback, helps avoid misunderstandings, and can clarify if the feedback given has been received as intended.

Box 7.8 Questions to facilitate feedback from a supervisee

- What have you found more helpful or less helpful in our supervision so far?

- Is there anything that I could be doing more or less of to facilitate your learning?

- How have you found the feedback I have given you so far?

- What helps you learn best?

- Has anything that I've said been unhelpful or made you feel defensive?

- Can you suggest ways in which I could have addressed the issue more helpfully?

- Is there anything else that you would like to share with me?

Use of Measures to Support Feedback

Another useful method for giving and receiving feedback is to use measures of the SR described in detail in Chapter 4. In practice settings, these can provide a starting point for discussions about the SR from both perspectives. For example, supervisors can use the Supervisory Relationship Questionnaire (Palomo et al., 2010; see Appendix 1) or its short form, the S-SRQ (Cliffe, Beinart, & Cooper, 2014; see Appendix 2) to gather feedback about the SR from supervisees. The Supervisory Relationship Measure (Pearce et al., 2013; see Appendix 3) provides an opportunity for the supervisor to provide feedback to supervisees on the SR. An alternative is the Leeds Alliance in Supervision Scale (Wainwright, 2010), which can provide session-by-session feedback on the supervisory alliance including the approach to supervision, the SR, and the degree to which the supervisee found supervision helpful. Other useful measures include the Working Alliance Inventory (Bahrick, 1990) and the Supervisory Working Alliance Inventory (SWAI) (Efstation et al., 1990).

All these measures were originally developed for research purposes, although the LASS and S-SRQ were also developed specifically to be useful in practice. It should be noted that, owing to the hierarchical nature of the SR, it is possible that results of measures used to gather direct feedback in practice may be positively skewed. However, any variation in item scores, however slight, will give useful information and provide the opportunity to discuss aspects of the SR that may not have come to light in general discussion.

The measures that we have developed (SRQ, S-SRQ, and SRM) and the LASS can be downloaded from the the Supervision section of the website of the Oxford Institute of Clinical Psychology Training (www.oxicpt.co.uk).

Unsatisfactory Performance

There are times when a supervisor is required to identify poor practice. In a training SR this may involve the failure of a placement or training program. This is likely to be the most uncomfortable supervisory task which brings the inequality and power dynamic of the SR to the fore. As with all feedback, clarifying competencies and evaluation processes at the contracting phase and establishing a mutual collaborative SR goes some way to making the process more transparent and manageable.

Unsatisfactory performance normally falls into three categories: incompetence, unethical practice, and problems with professional competence. Incompetence is perhaps the least problematic of these areas because it suggests a failure to reach an agreed standard or competency, previously defined by, for example, the professional body or training institution. In general, although it is painful for supervisees, highlighting the lack of competence in a specific area(s) can be helpful in identifying the further learning required to achieve the competency. It is rare for a supervisor to suggest that the supervisee is unable to develop the skills and competencies for adequate professional performance although it is, of course, a possibility.

Unethical practice involves infringement of professional codes of ethics or conduct; for example, entering into a sexual relationship with a client would provide clear grounds for failure of a training placement or disciplinary procedures for an employee. Again, the criteria are relatively clear and transparent, and professional regulatory bodies or employing agencies are likely to provide clear procedures to follow.

The area that has perhaps caused most difficulty for evaluative judgment and decision-making, previously named "impairment," is now termed "problems with professional competence" in the United States (Elman & Forrest, 2007). This differs from incompetence because it refers to diminished functioning due to extreme personal stress. Elman and Forrest argue that the term "impairment" confuses the supervisory role, which should stay focused on competence, performance, and meeting a professional standard. Similarly, Falender, Collins, and Shafranske (2009) warn against the use of the term "impairment" as it suggests a diagnosis or disability that is out of the normal supervisory realm and could be viewed as discriminatory.

When dealing with poor performance, it is essential to raise any issues and concerns clearly with the supervisee as early as possible. It is also important to consult others, for example, seeking the advice and support of professional colleagues and of your own supervisor.

Gilfoyle (2008) proposes 10 best practice guidelines for managing poor practice:

- provide written standards or competencies against which performance will be measured (usually provided by the training or regulatory body);
- have written policies of procedures to deal with competency problems;
- follow procedures and document meetings;
- apply standards fairly and ethically, and follow due process;
- establish internal review processes and respect confidentiality as far as possible;
- stay focused on problems in relation to training or professional goals;
- design remediation plans in line with program or professional criteria and goals;
- consider safety for all involved;
- keep a written record of all interactions and decisions;
- do not delay in addressing problems.

The majority of competence problems can be nipped in the bud with early and effective feedback and by finding external support, if necessary, for any personal issues that need to be addressed. The tendency however, is to avoid difficult issues to the point that they become challenging and distressing for all to manage (see Chapter 8 for further discussion). In the helping professions, there can be a tendency to overvalue the supportive function of supervision and to minimize the feedback and gate-keeping role. This can be counter-productive. It is therefore important for supervisors to recognize their power and responsibility to act quickly in the best interests of all concerned.

Summary

This section summarizes our and several other authors' views on best practice in giving and receiving feedback (e.g., Bernard & Goodyear, 2014; Hawkins & Shohet, 2012; Hoffman et al., 2005; Hughes, 2012; Lehrman-Waterman & Ladany, 2001; Scaife, 2009).

- Ideally feedback is related to learning goals, objectives, or competencies, which have already been negotiated during the supervision contract (see Chapter 6).
- Feedback works best in the context of a safe, trusting, and respectful SR.
- Feedback is an integral and mutual process within supervision (Hughes, 2012).
- Feedback should be given in a manner that is:
  - clear and unambiguous, so that the supervisee knows the issue to be addressed and how to go about this;
  - owned by the person giving feedback: that this is their opinion and not a universal truth;
  - regular and as an ongoing part of supervision (it is not helpful to save up feedback to the point that the issue becomes challenging to address or remedy);

- balanced, including both positive and negative aspects, so that supervisees are aware of what they are doing well and what needs to be improved;
- specific—linked to an achievable goal or learning need or to a specific piece of work that can be acted on (based on CORBS; Hawkins & Shohet, 2012).
- It is helpful to base feedback on direct examples (observed or recorded) of the supervisee's work (Newman, 2010).
- Feedback about multicultural issues should be raised in the contracting phase and presented in a culturally sensitive manner (Burkard et al., 2014).
- Feedback is most likely to be effective if it
  - comes from a credible source (Lehrman-Waterman & Ladany, 2001);
  - the recipient is open to feedback—timings are important;
  - relates to the needs of the learner and is invited;
  - balances tentativeness and assertiveness, support and challenge (Scaife, 2009);
  - builds on success—notice small changes;
  - is clear and fair—avoids humiliation or shame.
- Self-assessment should be encouraged.
- Feedback about feedback should be encouraged—be open to learning and receptive to feedback yourself.
- Be aware that supervisees value honest feedback but are also fearful of it (Bernard & Goodyear, 2014).

Conclusion

In this chapter, we have defined and described different types of feedback as well as summarizing the theory and research in this area. Methods to support effective feedback have been outlined. These include effective goal-setting and contracting for feedback preferences, methods of structuring feedback, constructive challenge, and self-assessment. We have stressed the importance of encouraging supervisee feedback as a method of strengthening the SR. We have collated information on best practice in giving and receiving feedback. The take-home message is that mutual feedback is integral to effective supervision and most effective in the context of a safe and supportive SR.

Key Points

- Feedback is key to learning and development, and giving feedback is an essential part of the supervisor's role.
- Feedback is most effective when it is given in the context of a supportive supervisory relationship.
- Developing a supervisory relationship in which feedback is a regular and integral part of supervision and can be reviewed and discussed is important.
- There are several models of feedback that can enhance learning and practice.
- Feedback needs to strike a balance between support and challenge.

- Feedback is best if it is regular, timely, specific, objective, clear, consistent, credible in relation to the needs of the learner, and developmentally appropriate.
- Mutual feedback is important in the supervisory relationship, and supervisors should strive to create a context within which supervisees can give feedback on supervision and the supervisory relationship itself.
- Inviting self-assessment and identifying and challenging strengths are useful methods of feedback.
- Supervisors often find the evaluative aspect of their role most challenging and may avoid giving difficult feedback.
- Supervisees generally report that they would like to receive more feedback.

8

Preventing and Managing Difficulties in the Supervisory Relationship

The aims of this chapter are:

- to describe the typical causes of problems in the supervisory relationship;
- to summarize how problems may be prevented in the supervisory relationship;
- to describe some options for managing difficulties in the relationship if they arise.

In this chapter, we focus on difficulties in the supervisory relationship—typical causes of problems and strains, the impact these have on the supervisee in particular, how to prevent them, and how to resolve or manage them if or when they arise.

Several authors argue that strain in the relationship in supervision is inevitable. The SR is a complex relationship that has an inherent power differential. The supervisee is expected to be receptive to feedback and evaluation, to be open to learning, and to try new things in order to develop as a practitioner. The supervisor is expected to provide support for the supervisee but also to act as evaluator and gate-keeper, and these roles may conflict (Mueller & Kell, 1972). Some suggest that conflict in all relationships is the norm and that, if it is resolved, can lead to stronger relationships (Farmer, 1987). However, it is often assumed that all conflict is negative. The SR can provide an opportunity for addressing and resolving conflict and for modeling conflict management in relationships at work. This may reflect a similar process to the tear-and-repair process highlighted as important in the management of ruptures in the therapeutic relationship (e.g., Safran & Muran, 2001).

Potential Causes for Conflict in the Supervisory Relationship

The multiple factors that influence the effectiveness of the SR have been discussed in detail in Chapter 3, and there are consequently multiple causes of conflict in the supervisory relationship. The challenges in the agencies in which we work cannot be overlooked. Many of us face high demands in our service contexts. We may be part of teams under stress, and have colleagues with whom we have

Effective Supervisory Relationships: Best Evidence and Practice, First Edition.
Helen Beinart and Sue Clohessy.
© 2017 John Wiley & Sons Ltd. Published 2017 by John Wiley & Sons Ltd.

dual relationships and little time for processing conflict or misunderstandings. Supervisors may have stressful experiences in their personal lives that influence their capacity to supervise (Clohessy, 2008). Power struggles are not uncommon in conflictual SRs (M. L. Nelson & Friedlander, 2001). Supervisors may have unrealistic, inappropriate, or unclear expectations of their supervisees, or feel anxious or lack experience about the evaluative and gate-keeping functions inherent in the supervisor role. This may be particularly relevant for newer supervisors who may lack confidence in their own abilities in this role, or the skills to manage power effectively. This may lead to the potential misuse of power and result in boundary infringements or poor ethical practice, which have been highlighted as particularly damaging to the SR (Falender & Shafranske, 2004; M. L. Nelson & Friedlander, 2001). Boundary infringements include dual relationships, which can be confusing for the supervisee and can create difficulties in the relationship, for example, if the supervisor tries to develop a friendship with the supervisee or to treat the SR as a therapy relationship (M. L. Nelson & Friedlander, 2001). Mismanaging the power differential in the SR, particularly in the context of cultural factors such as gender, ethnicity, age, and experience can also have a detrimental impact (e.g., M. L. Nelson & Friedlander, 2001), as can poor communication between supervisor and supervisee. Supervisors may not develop an adequate psychological contract for the relationship to establish mutual expectations, or may be perceived as lacking investment in the SR (Clohessy, 2008; M. L. Nelson & Friedlander, 2001) or as unreliable by the supervisee (Mueller & Kell, 1972). Supervisees may be over- or under-confident about their skills, and may feel overwhelmed by the demands of the service or by evaluation anxiety and consequently be unable to share or disclose their uncertainties about their work. They may adopt a defensive stance about feedback or be unable to develop or demonstrate the requisite competencies for their job, or even engage in unethical or unprofessional behavior. Table 8.1 summarizes some of the potential causes of strain in the SR.

Table 8.1 Summary of potential causes of problems in the supervisory relationship.

Supervisor factors	Supervisee factors	Relational factors	Agency/context demands
Failure to clarify expectations	Over- or under-confidence	Mismanaging power differentials	High demands for service delivery and paperwork
Inappropriate expectations	Defensiveness/ inability to respond to feedback	Lack of explicit psychological contract	Lack of clear expectations
Supervisor gate-keeping anxiety	Lack of investment	Mutual anxiety about evaluation	Dual relationships and conflicted teams
Lack of investment	Inability to manage service demands	Poor communication	Lack of time for processing conflicts and misunderstandings
Lack of confidence	Unwillingness to share evaluation anxiety		
Burnout	Inadequate competency development or ethical/professional violations		
Personal stressors			

Impact of Difficulties in Supervision and the Supervisory Relationship

The impact of difficulties in the supervisory relationship and supervision in general should not be underestimated. Research has shown that such difficulties can have a negative impact on supervisee well-being and health (Kozlowska, Nunn, & Cousens, 1997b; M. L. Nelson & Friedlander, 2001), their experience of training and future career goals (Ramos-Sánchez et al., 2002), their ability to work well with clients, their therapeutic relationships, and their experience of self-doubt (M. L. Nelson & Friedlander, 2001; Ramos-Sánchez et al., 2002). Unsurprisingly, such difficulties are associated with supervisees' reduced satisfaction with supervision (Ramos-Sánchez et al., 2002). Given that one of the purposes of supervision is to ensure best treatment for clients, what is of concern is that there is a reduced ability to manage adverse client-related events (Kozlowska et al., 1997a), and an avoidance of supervision and help-seeking (Kozlowska, Nunn, & Cousens, 1997a).

Although there is some research, more is needed about the impact of difficulties in the SR on the supervisee, particularly dyadic studies employing more objective measures of the impact on supervisees and on clients, rather than a reliance on supervisee self-report (Veach, 2001). Interestingly, there is no published research as yet into the impact of difficulties in the SR on supervisors. Our experience of working with many supervisory dyads and training supervisors from a range of professions, as well as our research in this area, suggests that difficulties in the SR have a negative impact on supervisors too. Many supervisors find them stressful, think about them a great deal, and, if the difficulties remain unresolved, they may lead to a reluctance to supervise in the future. Some research in this area would be a useful addition to the literature.

The onus on managing problems in the supervisory relationship tends to rest with supervisors. Research suggests that supervisees expect their supervisors to take responsibility for identifying and addressing any difficulties in the SR (Gray, Ladany, Walker, & Ancis, 2001; Moskowitz & Rupert, 1983). However, if supervisors ignore or mishandle conflict, this can lead to harmful and negative events in supervision (Gray et al., 2001; M. L. Nelson & Friedlander, 2001). Given that problems in the SR are not uncommon, can they be prevented? And how can they best be managed/resolved? Box 8.1 illustrates a case vignette of a problematic SR to which we will refer throughout this chapter to illustrate the principles of managing difficulties in the SR.

Preventing Problems in the Supervisory Relationship

At the heart of preventing problems in supervision and the SR is establishing a strong SR. Supervisors can do this by investing time in their relationship with their supervisee, particularly at the beginning (Clohessy, 2008). Establishing clear boundaries and expectations for the relationship through effective contracting (see Chapter 6) can also help to prevent problems by limiting the possibility of misunderstandings. And, of course, it's important to review this contract

---

Box 8.1 Case vignette

Sarah's view

Sarah is a new supervisor working in a busy inpatient unit. She has been asked to supervise Ben, an older male counseling psychologist approaching the end of his training who is looking for some experience of working within a particular thera-peutic model. Sarah is relatively new to the supervisory role. She has supervised a trainee once before, and is keen to supervise again. However, she is busy dealing with a number of additional responsibilities as a result of reorganization in the team.

Ben seems self-assured, confident, and aloof, and tells Sarah at length about his previous experience as a nurse on an inpatient psychiatric ward. He seems to want to focus on his clinical work from the first meeting, and they do not spend much time on contracting other than the pragmatics of how frequently and where they will meet for supervision. Sarah feels somewhat intimidated by Ben, as he is very different from her last trainee and seems much more confident. Early supervision sessions seem to revolve around Ben telling Sarah about his experience and how well things are going with his current caseload. Supervision often ends 10–15 minutes early, and Sarah feels unsure what she can offer him. She does not think she has a good understanding of Ben's learning needs as he seldom brings up issues with which he is struggling. She is aware that she will need to evaluate his competence and starts to become increasingly frustrated, so tries to exert more control in supervision sessions, for example by insisting that he bring recordings of his clinical sessions to supervision or that she sit in and observe him with clients. There always seems to be a valid reason why Ben is unable to follow up on these suggestions, however, and Sarah's frustration turns to apathy and she starts to give up on the SR with Ben.

Ben's view

Ben is nearing the end of his training as a counseling psychologist and is keen to develop his skills in cognitive behavior therapy. He has a lot invested in his train-ing as this is his second career, and he believes that he should be working much more autonomously at this stage. Indeed, his previous supervisors encouraged this approach. He feels nervous and is keen for Sarah to understand the skills and expertise he brings to his work, particularly given that he is returning to an envi-ronment he is very familiar with, albeit in a different role. He is anxious about recording sessions and is somewhat alarmed when Sarah suggests this. He does not feel safe enough to explore this with her, and feels she is somewhat unpredict-able in supervision –either over-controlling or uninterested in his work. He is very conscious that she will be evaluating him formally, and as such shares as little of his work with her as possible, only telling her the things he is pleased about.

---

and the SR regularly. The use of measures such as the SRQ or S-SRQ and/or a session-by-session measure such as the LASS (Wainwright, 2010; described in Chapter 4) to review the SR and the supervision provided may also help to prevent difficulties in the relationship. It keeps the relationship in mind, and the meta-communication is that the SR is open to discussion, review, and change. The supervisor can set the tone for the relationship by encouraging an ethos of learning from mistakes, by normalizing anxiety, and by cultivating a culture of openness within the relationship. Being clear and specific about the supervisee's strengths can also be important. Providing regular feedback to the supervisee on both strengths and areas for development, so that there is no ambiguity about their progress, can help to build confidence and a relationship in which the supervisee feels valued. This is particularly important for supervisees in training who are looking to the supervisor for summative feedback and evaluation. As well as providing regular feedback, it is important that the supervisor invites feedback from the supervisee. The power differential inherent in the SR may make it difficult for the supervisee to give feedback openly to the supervisor, particularly in training relationships when the supervisee is reliant on the supervisor for a positive evaluation. However, supervisors who invite feedback communicate a message that they are interested in the supervisee's experience of supervision and the SR, and keen to hear their views so that they can adapt as necessary. Self-reflection about how a supervisee may experience supervision with you as a supervisor can also be beneficial. Are you over-committed? Are you limited in the time you can give to the supervisee? Do you have issues in your personal life that may make you seem preoccupied? Reflecting on how the supervisee may experience supervision with you as a supervisor can help you to tune into potential conflict in the relationship. M. L. Nelson et al. (2008) suggest that wise supervisors remain self-aware and accept their own shortcomings.

Research suggests that both supervisees and supervisors need to remain open to the challenging aspects of learning, and that supervisors should maintain a stance of "openness to conflict" (M. L. Nelson et al., 2008, p. 177; see also Clohessy, 2008). This means that supervisors should be aware that there may well be conflict within the relationship, and alert for signs of this rather than assume that the relationship will be conflict-free. Ladany et al. (2005) describes these signs as conflict markers. In our research (Clohessy, 2008) a number of factors that could indicate a problem and potential supervisor interventions were identified. These included paying attention to both verbal and non-verbal communication, noticing and reflecting on reactions to supervision and the supervisee (e.g., tiredness, anxiety, working too hard), feedback from colleagues, the quality and length of the supervision session, as well as comparing the current SR with past relationships with supervisees. The importance of monitoring one's own emotional reactions to supervision and the supervisee can be a valuable source of information and is advocated in some supervision models (e.g., Hawkins & Shohet, 2012). Safran and Muran (2001) suggest the importance of tuning into the interpersonal pull in the therapeutic relationship, which may also be of relevance in the SR. This might mean reflecting on the behaviors the supervisor feels drawn to carry out in relation to the supervisee, for example, working excessively hard in preparing for supervision with the supervisee, feeling anxious or irritated, avoiding challenging the supervisee. It is important for the supervisor to reflect on how much these reactions are typical for them, and how much they are unique for this particular SR. Supervisors can make use of self-reflection

---

Box 8.2 Summary of preventing difficulties in the SR

- Establish a strong SR:
  - invest in the relationship and the supervisee—be interested in them, commit time and attention;
  - establish clear mutual expectations and boundaries through contracting for the SR;
  - review the contract regularly—check in to see how things are going;
  - encourage an open, collaborative ethos in which anxiety is normalized and mistakes are to be learned from;
- be clear about supervisee's strengths and give this feedback regularly;
- give constructive feedback regularly and invite feedback yourself;
- reflect on how the supervisee may experience you—be aware of your own shortcomings;
- remain open to the possibility that the relationship could become strained and look for signs that it's not going well;
- reflect on your own experience of supervision with the supervisee and any interpersonal pull you may experience.

---

or their own supervision for this purpose. Box 8.2 summarizes ways in which problems in the SR may be prevented.

Managing Difficulties

Research suggests that early detection of difficulties in the SR is important, particularly in training relationships, which may be of relatively short duration (Clohessy, 2008). Retaining a stance of openness to conflict (M. L. Nelson et al., 2008) and regularly tuning into the relationship for conflict markers (Clohessy, 2008; Ladany et al., 2005) allows the supervisor to spot difficult issues early, when there may be a better chance of resolving them. Research suggests that problems in the supervisory relationship are more likely to be managed successfully if *both* parties are able to consider their own contributions to the difficulty, and can discuss them non-defensively (Borsay, 2012; Moskowitz & Rupert, 1983). How we manage conflict in relationships is likely to be determined by a multitude of factors, including cultural influences such as gender (see Farmer [1987] for an interesting discussion of the factors that influence conflict management). An ability to use a variety of conflict management styles with some degree of flexibility is considered to be adaptive in managing difficulties in the SR (Farmer, 1987), with a particular emphasis on employing a collaborative style to maximize the potential to learn from conflict to develop the SR.

Opportunities to reflect on the SR can be helpful. The reader is invited to try out the questions in the reflective exercise in Box 8.3 (adapted from guidance on "Managing Difficulties" from the Oxford Institute of Clinical Psychology Training). In the example of the difficult SR described in Box 8.1, Sarah used the questions in Box 8.3 to reflect on the difficulties she was having in her SR with Ben.

Box 8.3 Self-reflection on difficulties in the SR

- What's telling you there's a problem? What are the markers?

- What are your ideas about the issue?

- What might you be contributing to the difficulty?

- What might the supervisee be contributing to the difficulty?

- Are there other factors contributing to the problem?

- What would need to change in order for the SR to work well?

- Are there any ideas that might be holding you back from raising it with the supervisee?

- Who could think the through the issues with you?

This helped her to clarify her thinking about the issues and prepared her to address the problems in the SR (Box 8.4).

The empirical research in the area of managing difficulties is limited, although there are some helpful practitioner guides (e.g., Ladany et al., 2005). Recent qualitative research has examined how experienced expert supervisors manage difficulties. In two studies of experienced supervisors in the United States (M. L. Nelson et al., 2008) and Australia (Grant, Schofield, & Crawford, 2012), a number of strategies for resolving difficulties in supervision were identified. Experienced supervisors were more likely to normalize potential conflict, to approach rather than avoid or deny difficulties (even if this caused discomfort), to give difficult feedback without shaming the supervisee, and to use humor, humility, and appropriate self-disclosure. Grant et al. (2012) found that experienced Australian supervisors used a number of strategies including relational, reflective, confrontative, and avoidant interventions to manage difficulties. Relational interventions were most commonly used, and involved the use of therapeutic relational skills such as empathy in the SR. Reflective interventions involved conceptualizing and understanding various processes in the SR as well

---

Box 8.4 Sarah's self-reflection

What's telling you there's a problem? What are the markers?
Feeling frustrated in supervision.
Ben doesn't seem to bring me the things he's struggling with in his work.
I wonder if he's avoiding bringing recordings of his work. It never seems to happen.
Supervision seems to finish early. Never experienced this before!

What are your ideas about the issue?
Is he anxious about his work but doesn't feel able to tell me?
He has lots of prior experience—is it hard for him to be in a (vulnerable) learning position? Is he not sure what I can offer him?

What might you be contributing to the difficulty?
Have I given up trying to make things better? Have I got the resources to try to work on this?

What might the supervisee be contributing to the difficulty?
Is Ben being as open as he could be? Is he making use of me?

Are there other factors contributing to the problem?
Busy context. Pressure to just get on with the work?
Gender, age, relative experience, power?

What would need to change in order for the SR to work well?
Full supervision hour to be used. Listen to recordings of his work.
For him to bring me the parts of his work he finds challenging as well as the things that are going well.

Are there any ideas that might be holding you back from raising it with the supervisee?
Worry that he might not rate me as a supervisor. It might make things worse.

Who could think the through the issues with you?
Discuss it with my supervisor. Practice how to raise the issue with Ben.

---

as monitoring what was happening. Confrontative interventions, including challenging the supervisee directly, tended only to be used by supervisors when reflective or relational strategies did not work. Avoidant interventions (e.g., withdrawing, denying, awaiting external intervention) were least frequently reported by this sample, and were used only if difficulties in the SR became too entrenched.

In Clohessy's (2008) study the supervisor's investment in the SR and the supervisee's openness to learning were highlighted as important contextual factors in the successful resolution of difficulties. If these factors were in place, the chance of resolution was improved. If they were not in place, the chance of successful resolution was reduced. The context of time was also important. The training placements described in this study were usually of six months' duration, so there was limited time to identify and resolve problems. Initially, supervisors needed to be aware of a problem in the relationship. Once they were able to identify a problem, they gathered more information, for example, provisionally checking things out with the supervisee, using their own supervision, or asking colleagues for information. Formulating and making sense of the problem was an important part of trying to resolve difficulties. Once the supervisor had made sense of the problem to some degree, they tried to raise the issue and made attempts to try to resolve it. Interventions were diverse, and attempts to resolve problems often provided additional information for the formulation. The supervisor needed to tune into the SR to see whether attempts at resolution were successful. If they were, the supervisor continued to invest in making the relationship work well. Successful resolution depended on the collaboration of supervisor and supervisee, on the latter's ability to remain open to learning, and on the supervisor's continued investment in the SR. Supervisors and supervisees could become stuck in the resolution cycle; for example, when the supervisor becomes aware of a strain in the relationship but is unable to gather additional information to formulate the problem (e.g., if the supervisee is not open about personal stressors influencing their ability and performance), or when attempts at intervention are unsuccessful (e.g., if the supervisee is not open to feedback and learning). If attempts at resolution are unsuccessful, supervisors may stop investing in the SR, and wait until the relationship reaches its natural conclusion at the end of the training placement. Figure 8.1 illustrates this model. If the supervisor stops investing in the relationship and the supervisee is not open to learning, the problem may remain unresolved and the supervisor and supervisee may become stuck in the resolution cycle, if they enter it all.

Formulation and making sense of the difficulty is an important part of the process of resolving difficulties. What models can we draw on to make sense of conflict? Any of the models of supervision or the SR (discussed in Chapter 2) can

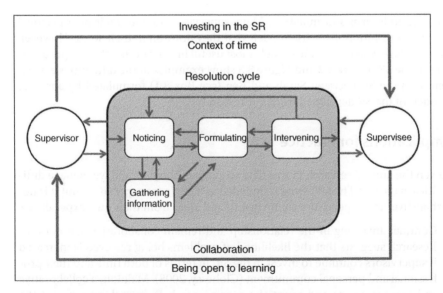

Figure 8.1 Resolving difficulties in the supervisory relationship. (Clohessy, 2008)

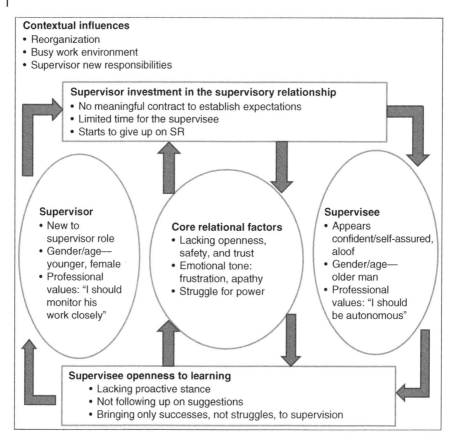

Figure 8.2 Formulating Ben & Sarah's supervisory relationship using Clohessy's (2008) model of the SR.

be used to inform a formulation. Many supervisors look to their own personal resources or intuition, or use models that they draw on in their work. However, we find supervision-specific models most useful in considering the unique qualities of the SR. Figure 8.2 and Figure 8.3 show examples of the difficulties experienced in the SR between Sarah and Ben (see Box 8.1) formulated by applying models of the SR developed from our research.

Implications for Practice

Given the limited research in this field to guide us, how should we manage difficulties in the SR? The following is intended as a guide for supervisors but it is not exhaustive, and supervisors are invited to add ideas from their own experience.

- Continue investing in the relationship and remain collaborative and curious. Research suggests that the likelihood of problems being resolved is increased if supervisors continue to invest in the SR, in terms of both time and their professional and personal commitment (Clohessy, 2008). Maintain a collaborative and curious stance and invite the supervisee's help in making sense of the

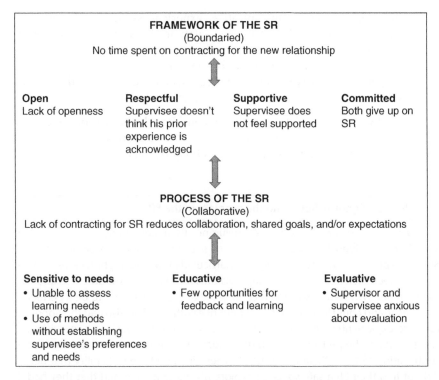

Figure 8.3 Formulating Ben and Sarah's supervisory relationship using Beinart's (2002) model of the SR.

difficulty and its resolution. This may be challenging, as strains in the SR can be stressful for both parties and there may be a tendency to withdraw or to bide time (Borsay, 2012; Clohessy, 2008; Grant et al., 2012).

- Tune into the relationship regularly and invite feedback from the supervisee about the SR; normalize conflict. If there is strain in the relationship, use your own supervision to reflect on this and to explore your ideas about it.
- Approach rather than avoid conflict. Use relational strategies to raise the issue with the supervisee with care and respect. Own your own contribution to any strain in the SR. Be tentative and curious.
- Formulate as a means of making sense of the difficulty. Once a strain in the SR has been noticed, you may hold a number of hypotheses and be able to tentatively check these out with the supervisee. You may be able to use one of the models presented in Chapter 2 in this process.
- If there is a rupture in the SR, use meta-communication about the rupture— step *outside* the process to communicate *about* the process (Katzow & Safran, 2007), particularly if communication becomes heated or fraught.
- Once you have developed a formulation, this should inform the choice of strategies you use to repair a rupture or to strengthen the relationship. Strategies for repair could include:
  - clarifying any misunderstandings that may have developed;
  - reflecting on the problem together and acknowledging any part that you as supervisor may have played in the development of the difficulty;

– building on strengths and positive experiences—be consistent and reliable—and re-establishing trust and safety in the SR if these have been compromised;
– being clear about your expectations for the supervisee;
– bringing in a third party to facilitate reflection on the difficulty in the SR and considering the best ways forward may sometimes be helpful.

Occasionally, it may also be important to consider whether to continue with the SR, and whether a change of supervisor would be a more appropriate solution. This may be because, in making sense of the problem in the SR, it becomes

---

Box 8.5 Case vignette: Resolving the problem in the SR

Following some reflection on her SR, including discussions in her own supervision, Sarah decided to initiate a review of supervision and the SR with Ben. She was apprehensive about doing this, particularly that she might receive some negative feedback about her own supervision. However, she was able to explore this with her own supervisor, and recognized that she didn't need to be a perfect supervisor, and could learn from this experience with Ben. She also had the opportunity to explore how best to raise these issues with Ben in her own supervision. Her supervisor helped her to formulate some hypotheses on what might be contributing to the difficulties in the SR. These included the possibility that Ben did not find their SR a safe space to explore his uncertainties, and that they had not been able to develop a meaningful supervision contract. She was able to practice owning her own position, and to consider how best to avoid triggering a defensive reaction in him

In their next supervision, Sarah asked if they could spend some time reviewing how their supervisory relationship was working. Ben seemed surprised, but open to a discussion about this. She started by asking Ben for his thoughts on how he had found their supervision sessions. He seemed initially cautious about talking about this, so Sarah offered her own reflections on their SR. "I've been wondering how helpful you've been finding our supervision sessions. I've noticed that it has been difficult for you to bring recordings of your work, or to discuss the issues you are uncertain about. I have been wondering how safe it has felt for you to explore your work here?" Sarah went on to acknowledge that Ben had a great deal of experience in working on the ward, and that she was keen to help him continue developing his skills in CBT and asked Ben if there were things she could do differently in supervision to help his learning. She also asked if they could spend some time exploring what he was looking for in supervision, and what had worked more/less effectively for him in the past. Ben was able to talk about his discomfort about bringing recordings of his work to supervision, and some of his expectations that he should be more autonomous. This led to a discussion about Sarah's expectations and what Ben would find useful in supervision. Once they were able to start talking about their SR, and what might make it work well, they were able to establish a more meaningful supervision contract, and agreed to review supervision regularly to ensure things were on track.

apparent that there is a mismatch between what a supervisee wants or needs and what a supervisor is able to offer. It is also possible that, despite the best efforts of both parties, the difficulties remain and are having a detrimental impact or that one or both parties are unwilling to work together to resolve the difficulty. In such rare situations, ending the SR may be the most sensible solution.

Conclusion

Conflict is common in supervisory relationships, not least because of the complex nature of supervision itself. There is much that both supervisors and supervisees can do to avoid difficulties, but if they occur supervisees often look to supervisors to identify and resolve problems in the SR. This requires supervisors to adopt a stance of openness to conflict and to monitor the SR for signs of strain. Making sense of the difficulty through the use of models to formulate can help. Certainly, a mutual commitment to change and collaboration, and the adoption of an open and curious stance by both supervisor and supervisee, increase the likelihood that difficulties will be resolved. Indeed, such experiences may provide valuable mutual learning opportunities. A variety of strategies to resolve difficulties have been suggested in this chapter, the success of which will depend on the nature of the problem and the value of the formulation. A mutual commitment to making changes in the relationship, and a willingness by the supervisor to continue to invest in the SR, are also fundamental to successful resolution. However, there may be some instances in which, despite everyone's best efforts, the only feasible way forward is to end the SR. In such cases, external consultation may help facilitate this process, and both supervisor and supervisee should be encouraged to reflect on the experience and the possible impact on their future SRs.

Key Points

- Problems in the supervisory relationship are common because of the complexity of the relationship, and it is the supervisor's responsibility to raise and address them.
- There may be multiple influences on difficulties experienced in the supervisory relationship, including supervisor, supervisee, and contextual contributions.
- Problems can have a negative impact on supervisees' health and well-being, as well as a detrimental effect on their work, and lead to an avoidance of supervision.
- Supervisors can help to prevent problems by establishing safe, open, and collaborative supervisory relationships through investing time, establishing clear boundaries and expectations through contracting, and reviewing the relationship regularly, inviting feedback as well as offering it sensitively.
- It is important to tune in to the relationship regularly, to look out for signs of strain, and to be willing to approach rather than avoid difficulties.

- Formulating and making sense of difficulties; raising issues with care, curiosity, and respect; and being aware of one's own shortcomings and contributions as a supervisor are helpful in managing problems.
- It is important for supervisors to be able to access support to manage difficulties through the supervision of supervision.

9

Reflective Practice

The aims of this chapter are:

- to describe reflective practice and why it is an important part of supervision;
- to summarize methods that can be used to facilitate reflective practice in the supervisory relationship;
- to explore methods of self-care for supervisors and supervisees.

This chapter explores the meaning of reflective practice (RP) and describes definitions, frameworks, and characteristics that contribute to our understanding of this way of learning and supervising. We will then consider methods to facilitate RP in supervision and the supervisory relationship, and provide practical guidance including examples of techniques and approaches to enhance reflective practice. An important aspect of reflective practice is self-monitoring and self-care so that you are able to enhance the well-being of others. We discuss methods of self-care to build and develop well-being and resilience towards the end of the chapter. Throughout the chapter, we provide activity boxes with suggestions for self-practice to exemplify the concepts.

What Is Reflective Practice?

Reflective practice has become a cornerstone requirement for most professional training, and reflective capacity is regarded by many as an essential characteristic for professional competence. It can be quite a challenging concept to grasp fully, particularly for those who place a high value on empiricism. In the early days of our own profession, clinical psychology, the scientist-practitioner approach was dominant, but in more recent years the reflective-practitioner method has been built into competency descriptions and training requirements so that both are seen as equally important for learning and practice. It is now a requirement for learning in all the helping professions (particularly nursing and medicine), and is fundamental to supervision and continuing professional development. The essence of RP lies in the consideration of the process of how professionals learn from their experience, so that they can integrate new knowledge and make sound professional decisions or judgments.

Effective Supervisory Relationships: Best Evidence and Practice, First Edition.
Helen Beinart and Sue Clohessy.
© 2017 John Wiley & Sons Ltd. Published 2017 by John Wiley & Sons Ltd.

This may involve both critical thinking and understanding the influence of their personal beliefs and values in order to develop the self-awareness that supports self-monitoring in day-to-day practice.

Donald Schon popularized the term in his two key texts *The Reflective Practitioner* (1983) and *Educating the Reflective Practitioner* (1987). Schon (1983, p. 68) defines RP as "the capacity to reflect on action so as to engage in a process of continuous learning." He distinguishes between "reflection-on-action" and "reflection-in-action." Reflection on action is a post hoc activity and may include reviewing a piece of work, individually, in discussion with a colleague, or during supervision. However, Schon argues that professionals need to be able to make moment-by-moment decisions during their practice, for example by choosing to follow one line of thought or action rather than another with a client. This activity he called "reflection-in action." Box 9.1 provides a suggestion for you to reflect on your decision-making in a recent session.

This capacity to step back and take a meta-perspective or "helicopter view" during practice—to think on one's feet in order to make moment-to-moment decisions that inform practice—is the process that Schon refers to as "reflection-in-action." Schon's model argues that practitioners need more than theoretical or technical competence to be effective practitioners. He provides an explanation of how professionals make choices or engage in professional "artistry" when technique needs to be adapted to a particularly complex situation or client. Argyris and Schon (1974) introduce the concept of "double-loop learning" to explain how our beliefs, values, and assumptions affect our strategies and decision-making at work. They note that there is often a gap between what professionals say they do (espoused theory) and how they actually practice (theory in use). The pattern of theory directly translated to practice is described as "single-loop learning," or error correction. However, in their study of professional decision-making, Argyris and Schon (1974) found that most professionals apply critical

---

Box 9.1 Reflection on and in action

Consider a recent session with a client or supervisee.

- Make a brief note of your line of inquiry.

- How did you decide to follow that line?

- Were you conscious of the decisions?

- What informed your practice?

analysis or judgment to their work (double-loop learning). This is elucidated by the construct of reflective practice, particularly reflection-in-action.

Various other authors have contributed to our understanding of RP. Kolb's experiential learning cycle (discussed in Chapter 2) incorporates a similar construct to reflection-on-action as part of the learning cycle: concrete experience (perceptions or feelings), reflective observation (reflecting), abstract conceptualization (thinking), and active experimentation (doing). Part of RP also includes self-knowledge, which includes the capacity to think about what you bring to the work, your own values, beliefs, thoughts, and feelings. The significant influence of contextual factors such as social, cultural, and economic issues are discussed in detail in Chapter 5. This acknowledgment of the self, in influencing the lens or frame through which one reflects, is often termed "reflexivity" and has been used extensively in systemic writing (e.g., Burnham, 2005).

To some extent, RP could be seen as taking an open-minded stance toward learning and all its influences. Early authors in this field, for example Dewey (1933, p. 29), defined reflective open-mindedness as " the active desire to listen to more sides than one; to give heed to facts from whatever source they come; to give full attention to alternative possibilities; to recognize the possibility of error even in the beliefs that are dearest to us." This definition of RP includes the concepts of curiosity, of learning from our mistakes and being open to challenge and feedback. As we have seen in our discussion of SRs the capacity to be open, self-disclose, share mistakes, and learn from feedback are part of what makes SRs effective and is supported by the emerging evidence base. Possibly one of the reasons why RP has gained influence in the helping professions is the strong evidence from other areas (e.g., pilots, surgical teams) that examining errors and learning from mistakes can significantly improve practice (and save lives) (Vincent, 2010).

Scaife (2010, p. 4) defines RP as

> the process of thinking analytically about what we are doing, thinking, and/or feeling, both as we are doing it and later in review from an observer perspective that allows us to use ourselves and the wider value-laden context in the frame, and which may lead to changes in or consolidation of our practice. It is a process which can be engaged in without the need for the stimulation of particular incidents but rather involves an attitude of open-minded curiosity oriented towards ongoing learning based on any of our experiences that are capable of informing professional practice.

Scaife (2010) describes a range of characteristics of RP:

- It is an active, intentional process that goes beyond description or replaying a remembered episode.
- It is an exploratory process without a predetermined outcome other than to better understand or improve practice.
- It involves curiosity and openness to alternative possibilities and explanations.
- It requires stepping back and taking an observer perspective or a helicopter view.
- It involves critical examination, questioning, and self-evaluation to create possible explanations for experiences (even if these challenge existing views).

Box 9.2 Creating a learning environment for the development of reflective practice

---

Think about a time in supervision when you were able to reflect on some work you found challenging.

- What facilitated this?

- What did your supervisor do to enable you to reflect?

- What might have inhibited this?

- It involves making links between a range of domains—theory, research, personal experience (current and past), intuition, wider literature, and the cultural context.
- It is about personal meanings and may lead to a more conscious knowledge of previously tacit beliefs or assumptions.
- It may involve changes to practice (unlearning) and trying out new ways of thinking, feeling, and doing.

It is thus important to create a context for this open-minded curiosity within our SRs and to note that the descriptive retelling of a clinical episode is not in itself sufficient for effective supervision. The evidence suggests that poor supervisors spend too long on case-focused discussions and not sufficient time on supervisee-focused outcomes or on the process of learning (Inman & Ladany, 2008). The key issue here is that we need to create a learning climate within the SR that supports our supervisees in taking a step back to make sense of their own experiences rather than going through endless descriptive retellings of their work. The exercise in Box 9.2 provides an opportunity to think about learning environments that are conducive to reflection from a supervisee's point of view.

Hawkins and Shohet (2012) describe five capacities of reflective practice in supervision in their influential book *Supervision in the Helping Professions*:

- learning and unlearning: being aware of your own learning styles and patterns and expanding your repertoire to prevent, or address, getting stuck in unhelpful patterns;
- reflecting: creating space within supervision to reflect, both externally and internally, on relationships and the wider system;
- relating: developing rapport with a broad range of people, staying fully and deeply engaged within the SR, and introducing the possibility of change or a way forward;

- collaborating: having the capacity to listen and to explore ideas collaboratively in a way that creates new understanding, knowledge, and capability through working together;
- sustaining personal and professional resilience through support and positive appraisal and maintaining a sense of hope/optimism and a sense of balance.

The authors suggest that these capacities are essential to those who work in the helping professions, and are also needed to make the fullest use of supervision. In turn, it is the function of supervision to nurture and expand these capacities:

> in supervision we collaborate and relate in order to reflect on the relating between the practitioner and their client(s), in order to create new learning and unlearning, that both transforms the work and increases the capacity of the supervisee to sustain themselves in the work. *(Hawkins & Shohet, 2012, p. 26)*

This is a helpful definition of supervision that brings the SR to the fore, introduces the concept of active engagement, and flags the significance of RP for change. We would also add that at times it is also important to reflect on the SR itself, particularly when things are not going so well (see Chapter 8).

Developing Reflective Practice in Supervisory Relationships and Supervision

The cornerstone of developing RP is to create the optimal conditions within the SR to enable supervisees to feel supported in honestly reflecting on their work. In their review, Mann, Gordon, and MacLeod (2009, p. 610) write:

> The ability to reflect seems to be amenable to development over time and with practice, and in the presence of certain stimuli (e.g., small groups). It also appears that the learning environment can have an encouraging or inhibiting effect on reflection and reflective thinking. An important factor seems to be the behavior of mentors and supervisors.

We have discussed the importance of creating safe SRs throughout this book and the chapters on contracting (Chapter 6) and feedback (Chapter 7), in particular, discuss the significant contribution of these skills to establishing and maintaining a safe SR. It is important to acknowledge that supervision involves a certain amount of emotional exposure for both parties. The supervisee may feel vulnerable or may experience the supervisor as powerful or intimidating. The supervisor may feel anxious about being "found out" or not being expert enough to meet the supervisee's expectations. Often these relationships are set up in anticipation, as the result of a range of factors such as past experiences, relationship to authority, cultural patterns, and hearsay before the supervisory dyad has actually met (Borsay, 2012). It can be quite challenging under these

---

Box 9.3 Beginning supervisory relationships

Take some time to reflect on a meeting a new supervisee or supervisor for the first time.

- Note down your initial thoughts and feelings.

- What influenced these?

- How did they impact your beginning a supervisory relationship?

---

circumstances to set up a relationship that is safe and trusting. The exercise in Box 9.3 supports reflection on the early contributions to SRs.

Our research (Clohessy, 2008) suggests that one of the key elements to establishing safe SRs is to invest time in getting to know one another at the beginning. Watkins (2011b) discusses the concept of the real relationship in supervision and how important it is from the beginning of the SR to create a genuine and authentic relationship with your supervisee. There are a number of questions that may help this process (see Chapter 6) and judicious self-disclosure may also begin to address the power differential in the SR, and to create a context that facilitates RP. In our experience (and informed by our research), it is worthwhile to set time aside in the beginning phase of the SR to attend to each supervisee and learn about their past experience, their unique learning needs and preferences, and any concerns they may have. This early exploration of expectations sets a positive tone for reflective practice.

Learning Styles and Preferences

Supervisees will have their own learning styles and preferences (see Chapters 2 and 6). The use of a practical tool such as an adult learning questionnaire (e.g., Honey & Mumford, 1992) can help identify personal preferences and clarify areas that need further development. Kolb's (1984) learning cycle is helpful to keep in mind in supervision with reference to the development of RP, particularly how best to enable supervisees to explore the whole cycle—from having an experience to reflecting on it, conceptualizing, planning next steps in an intervention, and so on. Supervisors can use a range of questions to help supervisees to reflect on their experience, and ensure that they are using the full learning cycle. Being aware of a supervisee's preferences and learning needs can be informative for a supervisor, and they can use a range of strategies to support the supervise to expand their repertoire.

The questions in Box 9.4 may be useful in enabling supervisees to reflect on a particular piece of work. It can also be helpful for a supervisor to be aware of

---

Box 9.4 Using questions to reflect

• How did you feel during this work? What thoughts did you have at the time?

• When did you feel most challenged, and what did you find most challenging?

• What sense did you make of that?

• What did you tell yourself at the time?

• Have you been in similar situations before? Did this situation remind you of anything?

• What feelings are you left with?

---

their own learning style preferences as this can sometime explain strains within the SR. For example, supervisors with active or experiential learning preferences may find themselves irritated or frustrated with supervisees with reflective or conceptual preferences. Noticing a learning style mismatch may provide a useful entry point for a reflective discussion on the SR.

Enhancing Self-Awareness

The key to RP is being able to position ourselves in relation to the often complex nature of the work we do, whether it is in health or social care or in an organizational or educational setting. We need to be reflexive, that is, aware of our own influences on our practice. But how do we become aware of these influences when they are not always immediately available to our conscious selves? Certain schools of psychotherapy require every practitioner to undergo their own therapy so that they can explore the unconscious processes that impact their relationships. However, this is not available or necessarily desirable for all those entering supervision. There are a multitude of different methods for enhancing self-awareness and it is probable that our differing backgrounds, values, and cultures, professional as well as personal, draw us to different methods. It is important, therefore, to take a little time to explore our own attitudes and values and to consider where these originate from and what influence they may have on our practice. For example, I (HB) recently attended a funeral of one of my earliest professional mentors and had the opportunity during the service to reflect on her contribution to my professional development. What came to mind was that

---

Box 9.5 Key role models

Think about the attitudes and values that you hold about supervision.

- Can you note down your key influences?

- Can you remember your best and worst experiences as a supervisor or supervisee?

- Are there key role models that have influenced your practice (positively or negatively)?

---

she set the highest of professional standards and then proceeded to support me to achieve these in a way that was manageable and flexible enough to fit in with my own personal and professional capabilities. This resonated with some of the influences and expectations from my family of origin, "to make a difference." I hope that I, in turn, have been able to flexibly support my colleagues over the years to make a useful contribution in their professional worlds. We invite you to explore the influences of your key role models in Box 9.5.

Having Conversations about Culture and Difference

The importance of being culturally sensitive within the SR was described in detail in Chapter 5, as well as the increasingly strong evidence base regarding the contribution of cultural competence to safe SRs and effective supervision. However, our experience is that most supervisory dyads find it hard to broach conversations about culture and many supervisors have not fully brought their own cultural influences to the fore. The activities outlined in Box 9.6, Box 9.7, and Box 9.8 outline some of the methods we have found useful in our teaching and supervision in this area, and we invite you to take some time to reflect on your own influences. The theoretical bases of these exercises are discussed in Chapter 5.

Using Creative Methods to Reflect

Up to this point we have focused largely on verbal methods to support reflection, but of course there are a range of different sensory modes (e.g., visual, auditory, kinesthetic) that can enhance RP. There is a small literature in this field, for example Mooli Lahad's (2000) *Creative Supervision: The Use of Expressive Arts Methods in Supervision and Self-Supervision.* Lahad suggests that creative methods are particularly useful when supervision feels stuck. It provides an alternative way of gaining access to perspectives or beliefs that may not be immediately accessible via purely rational conversational means. Creative methods can aid the development of RP as they have the common aim of providing

---

Box 9.6 Beliefs about difference

Use the social GGRRAAACCEEESSS acronym (discussed in Chapter 5) to explore your own beliefs and attitudes to some areas of differences (Burnham, 2010):

Gender
Geography
Race
Religion
Age
Ability
Appearance
Class
Culture
Education
Employment
Ethnicity
Sexual orientation
Sexuality
Spirituality

- Which of the social GGRRAAACCEEESSS do you attend to most in your work?

- Which are invisible or unvoiced for you?

- Consider your current SRs—which are named and which silenced?

Box 9.7 Cultural exploration of a supervisory dilemma

Consider a supervisory dilemma you have experienced (as a supervisor or supervisee).

- Explore the influences of the Social GGRRAAACCEEESSS.

- Were any of these relevant?

- Does this add to your understanding of the dilemma?

Box 9.8 Cultural genogram

Draw a cultural genogram (a map of key influences—include significant family and role models) of your professional experiences and influences.

- Use the social GGRRAAACCEEESSS list in Box 9.6, explore your own cultural identity.

- How similar or different are your values from those of your family of origin?

- What were your influences in developing your professional identity?

- How has this influenced your SRs?

---

alternative or different perspectives or new information. However, they should be used with caution as they may or may not appeal to supervisees (or supervisors) and can lead to somewhat unpredictable results (Inskipp & Proctor, 1995).

The use of metaphor can be a powerful avenue into gaining insight into a person's values and priorities. For example, Sommer and Cox (2003) report on the use of a Greek mythology metaphor to enhance reflection on development within supervision. Supervisees were encouraged to develop their own interpretations of myths and used questions derived from these stories to explore their practice; for example, what kind of self-care tonics might your flask contain? when you look at your work from the perspective of an eagle, how does the landscape change? Environmental or gardening metaphors are often used to explore the SR. For example, Valadez and Garcia (1998) used the metaphor of the supervisor as the sun and the supervisee as a seedling. The supervisor's rays contain the potential for the seedling to germinate and grow but also, if they are too strong, to burn or damage the seedling. Metaphors are often introduced into conversations by clients or supervisees and can be developed through curiosity and careful questioning. For instance, a supervisee may describe their working context as a steamship and a supervisor may develop a range of questions to explore this further: Who is the captain? Who is stoking the fire? Who is the ship's cook? What are the waters like? What would it take for the ship to change course? A quick way of accessing this information is to invite the supervisee to draw a picture of their image, depicting the key people and environment. A common drawing method (e.g., Inskipp & Proctor, 1995) is to invite the supervisee to draw their client as a fish and to represent themselves in relation to the fish (particularly useful as this does not require great artistic skills). Similarly, pictures or picture cards can be used to explore different perspectives. Supervisees can be invited to select images that best represent

---

Box 9.9 Images and metaphors

Bring to mind an SR that has caused you to reflect (e.g., you may feel it is stuck or is not as effective as you would like it to be).

- Can you bring to mind an image or metaphor that depicts this SR?

- If you wish, draw this image or metaphor and add details of context and so on.

- How would things need to shift for this SR to work more effectively?

- Does using metaphor or drawing develop new insights for you?

---

particular issues or concerns, and to describe or explore their choices and their relationship to the issue of concern and, potentially, to one another through encouraging the cards to talk to each other (Lahad, 2000). Metaphors using drawings have also been used to encourage supervisee case conceptualization (Amundson, 1988; Ishiyama, 1988) and, in their review of the literature on the use of metaphors in supervision, Guiffrida, Jordan, Saiz, and Barnes (2007) found this to be a promising method to enhance case conceptualization. The exercise in Box 9.9 invites you to explore images or metaphors to reflect on one of your SRs.

Using Live methods to Reflect

Reflecting Teams

In some therapeutic traditions, particularly systemic, live methods of supervision are the norm. Over the years, a range of live approaches have developed including the use of a one-way screen with telephone consultation, a "bug in the ear," or a supervisor knocking on the door to share their reflections. The current trend in systemic work is the use of reflecting teams within sessions (Andersen, 1987). This involves a small team of colleagues working together with families. Normally one colleague takes the lead in the interaction with the clients and the team is invited to reflect in the presence of the therapist and the family. The intention is to tentatively introduce new ideas that may shift the clients' understanding of the issue and assist in the recognition that there may be many perspectives to the problem or process. The therapist and the client are also provided with the chance to reflect on the reflections, enabling them to build on new ideas in the here and now, rather than waiting for a subsequent session post-supervision (reflection-on-action). This is a method that can be quite helpful in providing a structure for supervision groups and allows participants to practice reflection-in-action as well as to generate a range of alternative perspectives and possibilities for change.

Role-play and Rehearsal

In CBT role-play and rehearsal are live methods recommended for the learning and practice of specific skills and techniques (e.g., designing a behavioral experiment or socratic questioning) A supervisor may encourage a supervisee to practice setting up a behavioral experiment by taking the role of the client in the supervision session in order to provide an opportunity for the supervise to reflect on the role-play, with the supervisor providing immediate feedback and further rehearsal if required. Although these experiential methods are recommended for both learning skills and reflective understanding (Safran & Muran, 2001), there is some evidence to suggest that in practice they are not frequently used and that there is a tendency to rely solely on reported methods of supervision (Beinart & Clohessy, 2016).

Using Technology to Reflect

There is increasing use of technology in supervision and, with our growing technological age and busy lives, supervision is increasingly conducted at a distance. Rousmaniere (2014) adopts the term "technology-assisted education and training" (TAST) to summarize the diverse range of methods used including telephone, video-conferencing, Skype, and many more. It is beyond the scope of this chapter to review the many new developments in this field—Rousmaniere (2014) provides a comprehensive review. However, it is worth highlighting the significance of these developments, particularly the increased accessibility of supervision for practitioners in remote or isolated settings, as well as the development of a new range of complex ethical and legal issues including confidentiality and informed consent (see Chapter 5). The impact on the SR is yet to be fully understood, and we shall discuss this further in Chapter 10.

The impact of technology on the ease of recording our work (particularly therapy sessions for those of us working in these contexts) and documenting supervision provides unique opportunities for reflection and direct feedback on the process of supervision itself. There is increasing evidence that close monitoring and client feedback can significantly improve therapy outcomes; for example, clinical case management supervision (see Chapter 4) utilizes therapy progress to drive supervision (Richards, 2014). It is considered good practice to bring recordings of client work to supervision in order to enable the supervisor to provide direct detailed feedback on the work rather than purely relying on the supervisee's self-report. As we saw in Chapter 3, supervisees don't always report on clinical mistakes, and the use of direct recordings in supervision gives the supervisor direct access to the work. Detailed feedback on supervision allows the supervisee and supervisor to reflect together on specific aspects of the work and provides the opportunity for the development of micro-skills. Similarly, recordings of supervision can enhance supervision of supervision. There are several methods that can be used to discuss and learn from recorded material, which aid the development of RP. One such is method is interpersonal process recall (IPR) (Kagan, 1984). The method involves live recollection of any interpersonal process and inquires into the subjective experience of each participant. Areas explored can include self-exploration, views of others, behavior, values and assumptions, social and physical environment, and hopes and intentions. Using this method in supervision, the supervisee (recaller) brings recorded material to supervision and controls the replay, stopping the recording whenever there is a section they wish to explore. The supervisor (inquirer) prompts the recall by using open questions and inviting the supervisee to consider their thoughts, feelings, and images at the time. The aim is to help the supervisee develop insight and depth of understanding in order to articulate their reflections-in action through reflection-on action. The supervisor may invite reflection by using a series of open-ended questions to explore thoughts or images (e.g., What was going through your mind at that point?), feelings (e.g., What were you feeling, or what was the client feeling?), behavior (e.g., Was there anything that you wanted to say or do? Was there anything that stopped you?), hopes or expectations (What did you hope or expect to happen next?), and so on. The use of a structured method such as IPR has several advantages—it places the control and selection of material firmly in the hands of the supervisee, and is geared to help the supervisee recall and make explicit their own interpersonal processes rather than depending on the supervisor's perspective. This has a potential impact on power within the SR as the supervisee has control of the session and the supervisor's role is purely to elicit information from the supervisee. Like many reflective methods, IPR has the capacity to elicit previously unspoken thoughts and feelings, and consequently may be unsettling for the supervisee. As with all methods of supervision, careful contracting and review need to be established to ensure a safe space to reflect.

Using Reflective Writing and Journals to Reflect

Reflective writing has become the norm within many professional training programs, and is often seen as useful in ongoing development of professional skill and identity. I (HB) ask all new supervisees to keep a journal of their thoughts and feelings in relation to their work. All my current supervisees have such busy and demanding professional lives that it is valuable for them to capture significant moments that they can bring to supervision. My experience is that those who keep a journal bring slightly different material to supervision, which tends to be more focused on their own reactions and reflections than purely on the work itself. The use of reflective journals gives immediate access to supervisee-focused outcomes and shifts from a solely client-centered focus.

Writing is one way of capturing our thoughts and feelings and making them explicit, so we can critically reflect and submit them to thoughtful examination. Its relative permanence (compared to thinking or experiencing) allows us, if desired, to return to the material again and again.

Carroll and Gilbert (2005) suggest that practitioners prepare for supervision by taking some time to relax and reflect with their notebooks alongside them. They suggest that they let their mind drift over recent work and note what immediately surfaces. They are encouraged to note what went well, was more challenging, was uncertain or anxiety-provoking, was enjoyable, and so on.

Making notes of these reflections then allows the supervisee to prioritize material they wish to bring to supervision.

There are many different types of reflective writing including poetry, creative writing, narratives from a range of different perspectives, journals and logs (see Scaife (2010) for a helpful and detailed review). The most common reflective written method in supervision and training is via reflective journals. Reflective journals are generally used in education to promote a reflective stance toward learning and to help students integrate theoretical and academic content with their own experience and practice. There are a multitude of different types and formats for reflective journals and little current evidence to suggest that one form is more effective than another. Some authors suggest that it is helpful to separate the description of an event from the reflection, and it can also be helpful to add an action column (Woodward, 1998). It is advantageous to set up a system whereby it is possible to add later reflections. This is not an issue if notes are kept electronically but may need consideration if paper journals are used. The expectation of keeping a journal, or requirement to do so, can often seem effortful and be perceived as another task to add to the "to do" list rather than as a useful method to deepen understanding of learning and practice. It is thus important to support the supervisee in keeping journals in a way that is most useful, manageable, and accessible for them. If supervisees are not familiar with keeping written notes, it can be quite difficult to get started. In these situations, supervisors may encourage their supervisees to be creative and to note down thoughts, feelings, or responses in any form, without worrying about structure or presentation. It is essential to be clear and, in the contracting phase of the SR, to distinguish between journals that will be assessed as part of course-work, journals that are private documents, and journals to be used within supervision as an interactive resource (Burnham, 2010). If a supervisory dyad wishes to share aspects of reflective journals, this should be negotiated carefully in advance.

Reflective writing can also be used to reflect on supervision itself, in addition to other areas of professional practice. Reflective journals on supervisory practice aim to promote a reflective stance toward supervision and to facilitate learning and self-monitoring. For example, a reflective log of supervision kept by a supervisor may include a range of topics such as experience of the SR, emotional responses to the supervisee, assumptions or values that influence the SR, models that inform practice, ethical issues, issues of difference and diversity, the process of contracting and feedback, a supervisee's or supervisor's learning needs, and blind spots, strengths, and challenges for a supervisor or supervisee. Supervisees can keep similar journals about their client work and/or supervision. One useful way of exploring the material is to consider it from alternative perspectives, for example those of supervisee, client, or manager. The exercise in Box 9.10 can be used to explore writing as a method of reflection.

Self-practice and Self-reflection in Cognitive Behavioral Therapy

In CBT self-practice–self-reflection (SP–SR) is a way of applying CBT techniques to one's self. SP–SR uses a structured method to write down reflections on personal issues or experiences that may influence practice. Bennett-Levy (2006) proposes a model, the declarative–procedural–reflective (DPR) model,

---

Box 9.10 Using writing to reflect

Write down a brief description of a current or recent SR.

• What are the qualities of this relationship?

• Note down one example of an effective supervisory intervention and one example of a less effective intervention, and what you learned from these experiences.

• Now write these experiences from the perspective of the supervisee (or supervisor).

• Compare and contrast.

---

that integrates the three information-processing systems. The *declarative* system includes conceptual, interpersonal, and technical knowledge. The *procedural* system includes when–then rules and how information from client and therapist communications is processed. The *reflective* system involves processes such as focused attention to enable the mental representation of subjective experiences and the capacity for self-awareness and self-reflection. SP–SR reflective writing is a structured process that links personal experience to the practice context using workbooks and learning communities or groups where written communications are shared on a regular basis (Bennett-Levy & Lee, 2014). In a recent study, Bennett-Levy and Lee explored the conditions that optimize the benefits of self-practice and self-reflection, and found that engagement and a feeling of safety with the process were beneficial. These findings are not dissimilar to our own findings with regard to clarifying expectations, investment, and establishing safety within the SR (see Chapter 4). Bennett-Levy, Thwaites, Haarhoff, and Penny (2015) have recently developed a workbook for practitioners to support this structured method of written reflections that consists of 10 modules for self-practice.

Looking After Yourself: Developing Self-Care and Resilience

We discussed the evidence regarding the buffering effect of supervision for work-related stress and resilience in Chapter 4. Supervision plays an important role in supporting staff to work in challenging circumstances, and can play a preventive role by increasing staff retention and reducing burnout. For supervisors to be able to deliver the needed support, they must also consider how to look after themselves and to develop their own resources. There are several methods that may be helpful in supporting supervisor resilience. These include prioritizing supervision, seeking supervision for their supervision, and reflecting and being aware of their own need for support or resources.

Prioritizing Supervision

There is a tendency in our busy working lives to rush from one activity to another without allowing sufficient time between the activities to prepare and reflect, and therefore we do not maximize opportunities for learning. Additionally, in public sector contexts, supervision is often considered less of a priority than client contact. This can result in time for supervision being squeezed between other activities and, at worst, not being prioritized at all. We frequently hear stories of organizations not providing sufficient resources – time and space (e.g., a suitable room) – for effective supervision to take place. This can place great strain on supervisors and make supervision feel rushed, unsatisfactory, and unsatisfying. If supervisors are under-resourced in this way, it is very difficult for them to then be in a position to provide resources to others.

One possible solution to this problem is to plan a little time both before and after a supervision session to reflect on the supervisee's needs and on supervision issues. Allowing yourself time to prepare, make notes, and reflect before and after a supervision is likely to enhance your ability to be attentive and available for your supervisee – qualities that we know enhance the SR. The sense of being fully present for supervision links with recent studies that explore the relationship of mindfulness to supervision (Daniel, Borders, & Willse, 2015). This study found that supervisors' self-rating of mindfulness predicted the quality of the SR from their perspective but differed from supervisees' rating of the SR.

Supervision of Supervision

Many of us begin to learn our supervisory skills through our own experience of receiving supervision. We are likely to have experienced a range of supervisory experiences and to select and adapt our own supervisory styles from a range of role models. Supervision, just like other aspects of professional practice, should be reflected on and taken to supervision. This involves supervisors organizing their own supervision for their supervisory practice. It involves a complex set of skills that may or may not be available within existing arrangements for practice supervision. Setting up peer support or learning groups can be a useful adjunct to reflect on developing supervision skills. We discussed models of supervisee development in Chapter 2 but there are also models that describe supervisor development. For example, Stoltenberg and McNeill (2010) propose a parallel model of supervisor development to the integrative developmental model for supervisees. New supervisors at level 1 tend to show high motivation and anxiety about getting things right, and to focus more on the self than their supervisees. At this level, the tasks of feedback and evaluation may be challenging.

Supervisors at level 2 tend to be more aware of their supervisees' needs and may experience fluctuating motivation because of the complexity of the task. Supervisors at level 3 value supervision highly and invest in supervision. They have developed a strong sense of their own strengths and learning needs, as well as being sensitive to their supervisees' needs. Heid (1998) conceptualizes changes along thematic dimensions that include developing a sense of identity as a supervisor and building confidence and autonomy in the supervisor role. A significant theme is learning to use the power and authority (including evaluation) invested in the supervisor role. Supervision of supervision provides the opportunity for supervisors to reflect on their SRs and to note any patterns or conflicts that may emerge. It also provides the opportunity to try out supervision models and techniques, and is particularly useful for new supervisors as they develop their own supervisory style. Supervision of supervision groups are particularly helpful as an adjunct to supervisor training programs because they provide opportunities to apply theory in practice and to try out a range of supervisory interventions, as well as exposure to the different styles and approaches within the group. This can demonstrate the different learning needs and styles within the group and the importance of flexibility and matching supervisory interventions to supervisee needs.

Reflecting on Your Own Needs: Developing Resilience and Self-care

It is inevitable that, when you work with psychological distress or complexity at an individual, group, team, or organizational level, you will experience some level of stress yourself. This applies to both supervisees and supervisors. Supervisors may be one step removed from the distress, but it is likely that they too will be practicing and, even if they are only supervising, they are likely to be hearing multiple distressing narratives from multiple supervisees. It is therefore essential to be aware of your own needs and signs of stress, and to be able to support supervisees to notice and attend to their distress signals. Most of us have familiar bodily or psychological patterns that tell us when we are stressed. Typically, physical sensations may be in the form of headaches, stomach pain, disturbed sleep, or tiredness. Psychologically we may find that we lose concentration, have intrusive thoughts and feelings, feel overwhelmed, or begin to avoid certain situations. These are normative responses to difficult or challenging work environments which can be exacerbated if there are also personal or domestic stresses. It is our professional responsibility – identified by most professional ethical codes – to notice and manage our own levels of stress and to ensure that we are sufficiently resourced to do a good enough job. You can explore your typical signs of stress in the exercise in Box 9.11.

We also need to be aware of how we can reduce stress and build resilience so that we can support others to do so. For example, I (HB) used to read for half an hour every morning before going to work as a way of resourcing myself for the day ahead. Similarly, many people find exercise, yoga, cooking, the creative arts, and so on to be useful ways of switching off and relaxing. Normally, talking through, processing, and making sense of dilemmas is an important stress release, and supervision is often used in this way – this is the support function of supervision. Some find personal reflective space, reflective writing, walking,

---

Box 9.11 Noticing signs of stress

Note down your typical stress reactions—physiological, psychological, and behavioral.

- Can you identify early warning signs?

- Do you typically take any action when you notice these signs?

Box 9.12 Building resilience

What do you find helpful in building your resources?

- Consider personal resources, e.g., exercise, time for reflection.

- Consider social resources, e.g., social support, sharing concerns.

- You may wish to draw a map or spider diagram to illustrate your personal map of resources.

- Are there aspects of your current work environment that prevent you from developing the resources you need or that impact on your sense of autonomy?

- Can you problem-solve, increase flexibility, or make small changes to increase your resources?

---

or other solitary activities helpful in processing and reflecting on issues. If we accept that the work environment is stressful, then part of the task of supervision is to build resilience in others. Resilience is the capacity to use personal and social resources to increase well-being and to overcome stressful events without experiencing undue stress. The literature on supervision and staff well-being discussed in Chapter 4 suggests that there are at least three significant aspects to building resilience: individual resources, social support, and a sense of autonomy. The exercise in Box 9.12 explores how you can build your personal and social resources. Effective supervision helps supervisees notice and attend to stress, and works toward building resilience in order to prevent stress building up. Much professional supervision addresses issues of self-care and self-protection in demanding working contexts. It is often individuals in senior and high demand posts who do not prioritize self-care for themselves, although they may do so for others. There are often very simple strategies that can increase resilience. For example, allowing time to plan the day ahead or blocking out space in a diary to reflect on priorities. Supervision is a significant resource that allows both supervisees and supervisors to stand back, reflect, and take a meta-perspective, and it plays an important role in increasing both individual and organizational resilience.

Conclusion

In this chapter we have considered, defined, and described reflective practice (RP) within SRs. We have referred to key thinkers in this area, most notably Schon (1983) and Kolb (1984). We have stressed the importance of establishing optimal conditions for RP within the SR. In their systematic review of 29 studies of reflective practice in health care, Mann et al. (2009) found that the most influential elements in enabling the development of reflection are a supportive environment (both intellectual and emotional) and authenticity and adaptation to individual differences in learning style. We have suggested some methods to achieve this including contracting, using questionnaires to explore learning preferences, and having conversations about culture and difference. A number of methods to facilitate RP have been presented including creative methods, live methods, the use of technology and recordings, and the writing of reflective journals. Additionally, we have stressed the importance of using supervision to build resilience in supervisees and, consequently, considered how supervisors can develop their own self-care strategies in order to be able to resource others effectively. For those who enjoy reflecting on and in practice, we have provided a range of activities to offer the opportunity to reflect on your own practice as well as to illustrate the methods or models discussed.

Key Points

- Reflective practice is fundamentally about learning from experience through self-awareness, considering multiple perspectives, and integrating new knowledge in order to inform decision-making
- There are several helpful models to support our understanding of reflective practice.
- Reflective practice in supervision can also build resilience and enhance self-care.
- Facilitating reflection on the multiple influences on practice requires self-disclosure in the supervisory relationship.
- It is necessary for there to be a safe space within which supervisees can openly and honestly reflect on their experience of their work.

- The willingness to reflect on practice in the supervisory relationship is also influenced by learning styles and preferences.
- Reflective practice is essential to ethical and diversity-sensitive practice.
- There are multiple means that can be used to support reflective practice in the supervisory relationship including verbal, creative, writing, and technological methods.

10

The Supervisory Relationship in Other Supervision Formats

This chapter aims:

- to provide an overview of supervision in other formats, namely group supervision, remote supervision, and the use of technology to enhance learning;
- to summarize the relational issues of supervising in these contexts.

In this book we have focused predominantly on the relationship between supervisor and supervisee in the context of dyadic in-person supervision. In part, this is because much of the research and general literature on the supervisory relationship is on the relationship within this context. It is also perhaps the most typical form of supervision. However, with ever increasing demands in working contexts, as well as technological advances, delivering supervision in different formats is becoming more common.

In this chapter we shall consider the supervisory relationship within different supervision formats, namely group supervision, remote supervision and the use of technology (such as the telephone, Internet, video-conferencing, and software that summarizes client outcome data), and the special considerations for the SR in these contexts.

Group Supervision

Group supervision is often seen as a cost-effective and time-efficient means of offering supervision. It has been defined as:

> the regular meeting of a group of supervisees (a) with a designated supervisor or supervisors; (b) to monitor the quality of their work; and (c) to further their understanding of themselves as clinicians, of the clients with whom they work, and of service delivery in general. These supervisees are aided in achieving these goals by their supervisor(s) and by the feedback from and interactions with each other. *(Bernard & Goodyear, 2014, p. 161)*

While supervisees may express a preference for individual supervision and it is often considered a more traditional format, there is limited evidence to suggest

Effective Supervisory Relationships: Best Evidence and Practice, First Edition.
Helen Beinart and Sue Clohessy.
© 2017 John Wiley & Sons Ltd. Published 2017 by John Wiley & Sons Ltd.

that individual supervision is superior to group supervision (or vice versa) in terms of training outcomes, but the literature is small (Mastoras & Andrews, 2011).

Advantages of Group Supervision

Group supervision can be seen as offering a number of advantages including providing opportunities for learning from other supervisees, multiple perspectives, and exposure to the diverse range of work brought to the group. Additionally, supervisors are able to observe their supervisees' skills via their contribution to discussions and feedback to their peers. The group context has the potential to normalize anxieties about the challenges of the work, and also provides an opportunity for group members to develop supervision skills themselves, depending on their role within the group. Additionally, the efficient use of time and resources can make group supervision an attractive option (Bernard & Goodyear, 2014; Ögren, Apelman, & Klawitter, 2001).

Challenges of Group Supervision

Group supervision can also be a challenging context in which to learn because of a number of additional variables in this format compared to factors that prevail in a dyadic supervisory relationship. Groups have a complex interpersonal component, with potentially changing alliances between group members (Prieto, 1996). The added complexity may be due to problematic group dynamics, poor boundaries, and a lack of similar investment by all group members. Additionally, there is the potential for experiencing shame, rivalry, defensiveness, and competition, and these may reduce the experience of safety and the likelihood of honest self-disclosure (e.g., Ögren et al., 2001).

Requirements for Group Supervision

Good working groups have certain requirements for both supervisees and supervisors (Proctor & Inskipp, 2009) which are summarized in Box 10.1. It is helpful for supervisees to be clear about the tasks of the group and to agree on how they will work on this together. Good "group manners" such as sharing the time and space in the group, actively listening to one another, and respecting the views of all members contribute to more effective group relationships. Group members need to have an awareness of their own needs as well as those of other group members and the capacity to tolerate feelings of competition and rivalry. It is important that group members share similar values, beliefs, and assumptions about their work while also being able to value and accept difference. They need to be able to disclose and share their dilemmas with each other and with the supervisor. Group supervision potentially places more demands on the supervisor. Supervisors need to have confidence in exercising their authority and power when required, in facilitating a reflective space in a group context, and in promoting a group climate that enables each individual to find a voice. It is important that supervisors have an understanding of, and an ability to manage, group processes so as to make supervision in this context meaningful. Supervisors can also encourage supervisees to reflect on how the group is working in order

---

Box 10.1   Requirements for group supervision (adapted from Proctor & Inskipp, 2001)

Requirements of supervisor

- That the supervisor facilitates a group climate that is safe and in which supervisees can reflect on their work and find a voice
- That the supervisor is clear about the tasks of the group
- That the supervisor is able to identify and manage group processes
- That the supervisor is confident in using authority and power when needed
- That the supervisor invites supervisees to reflect on how the group is working

Requirements of supervisee

- That the supervisee agrees about the tasks of the group and how they will work together, and is able to reflect and feedback on how the group is working
- That the supervisee has good group manners – sharing time, listening, and respecting the views of everyone else
- That the supervisee is aware of their own needs as well as the needs of others in the group, and has the capacity to tolerate competition, rivalry, etc.
- That the supervisee shares values but is also able to tolerate and accept differences

---

to get the most out of the experience (Boëthius & Ögren, 2000; Ögren & Sundin, 2007; Proctor & Inskipp, 2009).

Types of Groups

Proctor & Inskipp (2001) describe four different types of groups, which belong on a continuum, according to the role of supervisor and the contribution of group members. The *authoritative group* is described as supervision *in* the group. Supervision in this format is similar to individual supervision, with the supervisor supervising each group member in turn and the other supervisees acting as observers on the process. The *participative group* is described as supervision *with* the group. In this format the other group members contribute more to each other's learning, although the supervisor maintains the lead and monitors the task of the group as well as the individual supervisee and the group as a whole. In this format, group members also have the opportunity to develop supervisory skills as they contribute to each other's learning through offering their perspectives and giving feedback. The *cooperative group* can be viewed as supervision *by* the group and, while the supervisor retains overall responsibility, the running of the group is largely managed by the group itself. Finally, the *peer group* describes a format in which each member takes shared responsibility for supervision and acts as supervisor for the others, and in which the responsibilities for the group are negotiated and shared.

Defining these different types of groups is important to clarify the purpose, roles, and expectations of the group. A group will develop over time, and the way it is used by group members may stay the same for the life of the group or it may change and evolve. For example, the group may begin as authoritative (with the supervisor taking primary responsibility for the supervision and leading the group) and evolve into a more cooperative or even a peer group, as group members become more involved in supervising each other and monitoring the group itself.

In addition to clarifying the type of a supervision group, it is also important to consider its size and the optimal number of supervisees. Larger supervision groups may provide more opportunities for learning but also more chances for individual supervisees to hide in the group or for some members to become more dominant (Boëthius, Sundin, & Ögren, 2006). Groups of four supervisees have been suggested as optimal because they provide the opportunity for equal participation and the development of strong group relationships (Boëthius et al., 2006).

As mentioned earlier, an understanding of group processes is also important in facilitating group supervision, and we shall describe some literature in this area next.

Understanding Group Processes

Much of the literature on group supervision draws on the psychotherapeutic literature on groups, particularly understanding group processes and development. While therapy groups have different aims and objectives to supervision groups, the understanding of group dynamics that the therapy field offers can be helpful in the supervisory context. Learning in a group can be a powerful experience that can stay with the group member long after the group has ended (Ögren et al., 2001). The consequences of being part of a group can be both positive and negative, and an understanding of group dynamics can help to promote positive consequences and hopefully mediate negative ones (Ögren, Boëthius, & Sundin, 2014).

Schütz (1967) describes three basic needs of the individuals within a group that develop and change as the group begins to work together:

- *Inclusion needs*: In the early stages of group supervision, supervisees consider their position, including their experience of acceptance and belonging within the group. Supervisors can encourage supervisees to get to know each other and to model acceptance of each group member.
- *Power and influence needs*: As the group develops, members explore their own influence and power, which may result in some competition and power struggles. Supervisors need to manage this sensitively.
- *Affect needs*: As the group matures, members decide how best to work together, are open about themselves and their experiences, and accept their differences. Supervisors demonstrate empathy, acceptance, and genuineness, and facilitate the exploration of any group conflict.

It can be helpful for supervisors to be aware of these needs and to gauge their interventions in the group accordingly. In addition to the needs of the individuals within the group, some authors have suggested that groups progress through a number of stages that can impact a supervisor's role and relationships within the group. The group process model described here has been very influential in this area (Tuckman, 1965; Tuckman & Jensen, 1977):

- *Forming*: As the group begins, members work toward feeling more comfortable with each other. Supervisors facilitate this process by contracting and establishing rules for the group to enable a culture of safety and trust.
- *Storming*: Group members may compete with each other in an overt or covert way, and there may be a struggle for power within the group.
- *Norming*: The culture of the group develops through members working to establish acceptable behavior and, often, unspoken rules emerge within the group. Supervisors need to be aware of the group culture and of its unspoken rules, and to monitor its impact on individual group members.
- *Performing*: This is seen as the most productive stage of the group. It is important for supervisors to be open to feedback and to be generally supportive, particularly in this stage, in order to normalize mistakes and to model this way of interacting so that group members can feel safe in offering this support to each other and in disclosing their struggles with the work.
- *Adjourning*: This is the stage at which the group works on endings, takes stock, reviews and makes sense of the work of the group (hopes, expectations, and any disappointments), evaluates individual progress, and establishes an ongoing plan for individuals' continuing development. If it is not time-limited, scheduling in regular reviews can be a useful way of marking transitions for the group.

There is evidence that a sense of security is important in group supervision, just as safety is fundamental to individual supervision. A sense of security in groups facilitates openness and group cohesion, which can also mean that different opinions and perspectives are tolerated, valued, and seen as enriching (Ögren et al., 2001). Insecurity in groups can be characterized by lack of trust, safety, rivalry, competition, lack of group cohesion and support, and the formation of subgroups. Learning in such contexts can be challenging. Group composition can influence how group processes and the group climate develop (Ögren et al., 2001). A degree of homogeneity in groups is considered helpful. If there are too many differences between group members in areas such as maturity, experience, motivation, and cultural factors, these may interfere with the development of security within the group (Ögren et al., 2001). It is also important to consider what other factors supervisees bring to the group that may influence the group climate and processes. Pre-existing personal problems and a high degree of emotional vulnerability in group members may influence how able a supervisee is to tolerate the learning role, and their need for closeness and confirmation within the group. This could contribute to a more insecure group climate (Ögren et al., 2001). Some writers suggest that supervisees may re-enact previous patterns and roles from their earlier experiences in groups (such as their family of origin), which will also influence their participation in and contribution to the supervision group (e.g., Cooper & Gustafson, 1985). Finally, the organizational framework in which group supervision occurs will also influence the processes and climate of the group. For example, if the supervision group is part of a training program or part of the work context (Ögren et al., 2001), there will be associated demands, stressors, and agendas that will influence the group.

In summary, some knowledge of group processes can enable supervisors to make sense of group behaviors and relationships, and to intervene appropriately. It can also guide them in the relational tasks inherent in the supervisory role in group supervision.

Supervisor's Relational Tasks

The supervisor's primary relational task is to create a supportive and safe group context, but this can be challenging and may require a great deal of skill in both supervision and managing group processes. In a qualitative study, Fleming, Glass, Fujisaki, and Toner (2010) suggest that safety is facilitated by group cohesion, that is, mutual engagement in the group through sharing experiences and resolving conflict. Group facilitation that encourages supervisees to take the lead in initiating discussions and giving mutual feedback, as well as a willingness to explore the group process, are thought to be helpful supervisory interventions. Bernard and Goodyear (2014) suggest that supervisors are often more comfortable with the skills associated with the supervisory task than with the skills related to managing group processes, and that these may require differing skill sets and training.

Creating Safety in Groups

The primary purpose of supervision groups is to develop in such a way that there is sufficient cohesion and interpersonal trust to enable group members to explore their professional dilemmas safely (Bernard & Goodyear, 2014). The relational challenge for the supervisor is to establish and maintain multiple SRs with supervisees; to establish safety and trust within the group context, including the need for a secure framework and containing boundaries; to tune in to these relationships and monitor them for signs of strain or rupture; and to facilitate the establishment of helpful working relationships between group members. Competition and rivalry may develop between supervisees, and those who identify as different in some way (e.g., due to cultural variables such as age, gender, ethnicity, or sexuality) may choose to isolate themselves from the rest of the group or may feel ostracized (Ellis & Douce, 1994). These processes should be identified and addressed by supervisors to develop a more cohesive, mutually supportive group climate. It is important for supervisors to consider the relationship histories of group members. For example, have they worked together before? Do they share a working context external to the group? Sussman, Bogo, and Globerman (2007) suggest that this can influence the group, particularly if some members know each other better than others and have pre-existing professional relationships outside the group. Group supervisors, therefore, have the task not only of establishing and maintaining their own SRs with supervisees in the group, but also of tuning in to the relationships between supervisees and to the group process.

Contracting

We have stressed the importance of developing meaningful psychological contracts in individual supervision, and these principles are also fundamental in groups as a way of establishing safety and developing supervisory alliances.

Contracting should include discussion and negotiation about the purpose and goals of the group as well as the ground rules for working together effectively. Inviting the group to consider the factors that will promote safety, enable group members to share their work with each other, and facilitate collaboration between supervisor and supervisees can be very helpful. Supervisors can also invite discussion about factors that may impede safety and disclosure, such as competition with each other, anxiety, or avoidance. Educating group members about group processes can also form part of contracting discussions and provide the basis for inviting everyone to observe and monitor their own responses as well as those of the group as a whole. Explicitly acknowledging and valuing diversity and difference is also an important part of early contracting discussions with the group. See Box 10.2 for an example of topics that can be included in developing a group supervision contract. This is not intended as an exhaustive list but as a starting point for some of the key issues to include in contracting for the relationships in the group.

Just as with individual supervision, it is important for supervisors to share their expectations as well as the factors they value from their supervisory relationships. Supervisors can acknowledge that they are aware of the vulnerability involved in bringing work that is genuinely challenging to share with the group, and invite supervisees to consider how they might be supported by the supervisor, and each other, to take the risks inherent in doing this. It is also helpful for supervisors to share an enthusiasm for group supervision, and to be able to highlight the potential benefits of learning in this context.

A clear structure for the group is important, particularly early on in its development. It is helpful to negotiate this structure with the group at the contracting stage, for example, by considering pragmatic details such as how the group will run, how time will be shared between members of the group, whether group members will be required to bring audio or video recordings of their work, and expectations with regard to preparing for supervision to ensure that supervisees get the most out of the experience. Supervisors may be required to be active and visible in the group initially, depending on the type of group supervision offered. In this way, supervisors can help to influence and set the tone for the group climate, and to model active listening, respect for diversity and different perspectives, and the sensitive giving of feedback.

Giving Feedback and Evaluation

As we saw in Chapter 7 in relation to individual supervision, an important task for supervisors is giving feedback to supervisees. This can be a particularly sensitive task in group supervision (Sussman et al., 2007). Supervisors should be mindful of the capacity for shaming supervisees in front of their peers (or of giving excessive praise or criticism to individual group members) and of the potential impact their feedback may have on other members of the group (Bernard & Goodyear, 2014). It is important to create a climate of learning from mistakes and of encouraging supervisees to present work that has genuinely challenged them rather than selecting only "safe" work that casts them in a favorable light (Ögren et al., 2014). In group supervision, there are opportunities to learn from each other, to share different perspectives on the work discussed, and to receive

---

Box 10.2 Questions to facilitate the development of the group supervision contract

---

- What ground rules might we need to create a safe space in the group? (Consider confidentiality, respectful challenge, listening to each other, sharing the space, and valuing difference.)

- What has been your experience of group supervision in the past?

- What has been helpful or unhelpful in your past experiences of supervision generally (dyadic and group)?

- The things we value in group supervision are … (Consider supervisor and supervisee perspectives.)

- What are you hoping for from the group?

- What are our goals, both individual and as a group?

- What should we know about each other that is important? (An invitation to share aspects of professional practice and/or personal information.)

- How will the group run? Consider frequency, duration, and format of the group. How will the supervision be organized and the supervision space shared?

- What are our feedback preferences? How do we like to be given feedback?

- How might we notice and discuss aspects of the group process that impact supervision?

- How shall we approach any strains or problems that we notice or experience in the group?

- How and when do we review the group?

feedback from other group members as well as the supervisor. Sharing feedback preferences is an important part of contracting, and of course it is important to ensure that these preferences are respected. The supervisor also needs to consider the developmental needs of the supervisees in the group (which may be different) and will need to be flexible in the approach they use. As with offering feedback in dyadic supervision, this should sensitively identify and highlight strengths in line with a supervisee's preferences, and provide clear opportunities for further development (Anderson, Schlossberg, & Rigazio-DiGilio, 2000; Mastoras & Andrews, 2011; Sussman et al., 2007). Whether there is a formal evaluative component to the group supervision will depend on the type of supervision group and the organizational context in which it occurs. If the group is part of a training program, the supervisor and supervisees must be clear about the competencies supervisees are required to demonstrate, and how the supervisor will assess these. In group supervision, it is also important to consider what aspects (if any) of formal evaluation are shared in the group context (particularly in light of the potential for shame, competition, and rivalry) or whether this is kept to an individual format.

Dealing with Problems

Fostering trust, mutual support, and group cohesion have already been highlighted as important supervisory interventions in creating a helpful group climate. Creating this context may be important in preventing major problems developing in the group. However, despite a supervisor's best efforts to create a secure, safe working context, it may not be possible to achieve this and difficulties in the group may still develop. Many of the same principles on managing difficulties highlighted in Chapter 8 are applicable to groups, namely tuning into the relationships in the group (as well as the emotional tone of the group as a whole), developing hypotheses and making sense of any ruptures or difficulties, and a general stance of approaching rather than avoiding problems in the group. Supervisors need to tune in to the group climate, and notice markers that might indicate problems. There may be obvious signs of strain in group relationships, but these may also be less obvious, for example, there may be too much agreement or conformity amongst group members (Carlson, Rapp, & Eichler, 2012). However, there is arguably an added complexity in formulating and making sense of problems in a group context because of the need to factor in group processes.

Box 10.3 summarizes some factors to consider in making sense of difficulties that may arise in group supervision. Again, this is not intended as an exhaustive list but is rather some key factors to bear in mind when trying to formulate and make sense of problems. Some of these relate to factors within the group itself; often the first reaction is to look for causes of problems internally (Ögren et al., 2014), but difficulties experienced within the group may also relate to the context within which the group takes place and the processes at play in this wider context. Of course, it is also important to consider any contribution the supervisor may be making, perhaps to do with leadership style or their ability to create a safe and secure working context.

Box 10.3 Issues to consider in making sense of problems in group supervision

- Are any problems to do with the stage of the group (e.g., characteristic of group "storming" [Tuckmann & Jensen, Tuckman and Jensen, 1977])?

- Might the composition or size of the group be relevant (e.g., too much heterogeneity or too many differences between members)?

- Have supervisees been in group supervision before? Might their prior experiences in supervision be relevant?

- Are the goals, purpose, and function of the group clear?

- Have the ground rules been agreed? Is confidentiality clear?

- Is the structure of the group appropriate to the needs of supervisees?

- Are any problems related to individual supervisees' personal difficulties (e.g., a high degree of emotional vulnerability, an inability to be reflective or to take risks in the group, or a need to dominate the group space)?

- Are any tensions related to group members' pre-existing relationships with each other?

- Might any problems reflect processes within the broader context (e.g., the work environment or training program)? Is the broader context supportive of the supervision group? What is its agenda for the group?

- Might any problems reflect any parallel processes in the work presented in the group?

- Might difficulties reflect roles that supervisees have taken in earlier groups of which they have been part (e.g., their family)?

- What contribution might I (as supervisor) be making to the difficulties observed? Is my supervisory style a good match for the group? Am I comfortable in this leadership role? Am I too dominant or not present enough in leading the group? Am I investing enough in the group?

- Is the group able to reflect on the process of the group and to give appropriate feedback?

Once any strains or problems in the group have been noticed and considered, it is the supervisor's responsibility to address these. Their intervention will depend on how they conceptualize or formulate the issues. In the contracting phase, there should have been some discussion and agreement about how problems in the group will be addressed, and the supervisor may wish to invite the group to observe patterns and processes and negotiate how to manage them. Supervisees should be encouraged to take responsibility for the group and to contribute to making it work well.

As we can see, there are multiple and complex tasks for the supervisor in establishing and maintaining supervisory relationships in group supervision, but this modality can be rewarding for those involved, not least in helping group members to work together effectively and to support each other's learning. The group process itself can be used to facilitate positive supervisory outcomes and to consolidate SRs. Supervision is commonly delivered in person, and developing and maintaining SRs in these contexts is familiar territory for most supervisors. However, in recent years there has been an increase in the use of technology in supervision, and as such it can also be delivered remotely. The next section considers some of the relational benefits and challenges of SRs in these contexts.

Remote Supervision and the Use of Technology

Technological advances provide supervisors and supervisees with a number of different methods or formats to enhance supervision or increase the accessibility of supervision as a resource. Video-conferencing (such as Skype), use of the Internet or online resources, and routine outcome measurement software can all be used to enhance more traditional formats of supervision. For example, video-conferencing can be used to provide live supervision in place of more traditional (and expensive) one-way screens (Rousmaniere & Frederickson, 2013). This method of supervision is more common in some forms of psychological therapy (such as family therapy) and offers the advantage of providing opportunities for experiential learning, and "in the moment" feedback and guidance on the work of the supervisee. Similarly, many clinical services are using software that records and summarizes regular routine outcome measures from clients. This provides a more objective source of information on client progress and change, and can be used in supervision to guide discussion and prioritize which clients should be discussed. In terms of the supervisory relationship, supervisors should be sensitive to supervisees feeling particularly exposed using either live supervision or routine outcome software. Their practice can be scrutinized and feedback provided in greater detail using these methods, which is an advantage, but these methods also require a safe, supportive relational context in which the supervisee can take advantage of this and maximize their learning.

Advances in technology have also increased the use of remote supervision— that is, supervision that is not provided in the traditional face-to-face format, such as via telephone, video-conferencing, or online.

Advantages of Remote Supervision

Rousmaniere and Ellis (2013) highlight a number of strengths of remote supervision using a range of technologies. They suggest that it enables professionals to have access to a wider range of supervisors than may be available locally, which can increase the possibilities for learning and development. This is particularly relevant for those in remote geographical areas where the supervisory resource may be small and access to good supervision and professional support more difficult. Providing this via remote supervision may be particularly important in improving the services available to these communities, as well as in supporting the professionals working in these areas (Reese et al., 2009). Access to a wider supervisory resource may also be important in work contexts in which the politics of the organization makes access to safe, effective supervision difficult. Finally, remote supervision can also be advantageous if a degree of consistency is required in a service offered across a number of locations, for example, in research trials carried out over multiple sites.

The research on remote supervision suggests that it can be satisfactory to supervisees (Xavier, Shepherd, & Goldstein, 2007) and there is some preliminary research on the supervisory alliance in this area. In a small-scale study comparing group supervision provided both in person and via video-conferencing, Reese et al. (2009) found that supervisees were just as satisfied with their supervisory relationships regardless of whether they met in person or remotely via video-conferencing. Additionally, there is some evidence to suggest that remote supervision may promote self-disclosure (Cummings, 2002; Sorlie, Gammon, Bergvik, & Sexton, 1999) increase self-efficacy and reduce feelings of isolation (Panos, 2005; Weingardt, Cucciare, Bellotti, & Lai, 2009), and that both supervisors and supervisees may be more likely to prepare more thoroughly for it, which can also be seen as a helpful outcome (Sorlie et al., 1999).

Challenges of Remote Supervision and the Use of Technology

There are a number of challenges in using technology in supervision. Supervisors providing remote supervision may be unfamiliar with local professional practice or organizational regulations (Abbass et al., 2011) and have little knowledge of the cultural context within which the supervisee is working (Rousmaniere, 2014). Supervisors need to consider how to manage any concerns about their supervisee's competence and practice when they may not be familiar with the work or professional context under discussion. There may also be challenges related to the accessibility of the supervisor in an emergency. Arranging access to another back-up supervisor who is local to the supervisee, is familiar with the working and cultural context, and can take forward any concerns regarding supervisee competence, as needed, may be a helpful solution to these challenges (Abbass et al., 2011; Panos, 2005).

There are a number of ethical issues inherent in using technology in supervision, the most obvious of which is client confidentiality. There may be the potential for breaches of confidentiality in using video-conferencing software such as Skype or sharing data to the Internet cloud (e.g., through Dropbox or Apple iCloud). Using encryption software if sharing confidential information via the Internet, ensuring that privacy settings are set to "private," and taking steps to maximize security online (by choosing appropriate passwords, etc.) are all important in using technology safely and ethically in supervision (see Rousmaniere, 2014, for a helpful summary). It is also important to gain informed consent from supervisees and their clients (Rousmaniere, Abbass & Fredrickson, 2014).

Additionally, the use of technology requires a degree of confidence and competence with these methods that arguably places more demands on the supervisor (and supervisee), and supervision may feel like harder work. There may be technological problems, such as a loss of Internet connectivity which can interrupt and interfere with the work of supervision and be frustrating for both supervisor and supervisee. It is perhaps sensible to agree back-up methods of communication if the technology used does not work effectively (Rousmaniere, 2014). Finally, there may be some limitations in the variety of learning methods available for use via some methods of remote supervision (such as telephone supervision). Again, there is perhaps a case for ensuring that remote supervision is not the only means of supervision for the supervisee, and that it is augmented by other, more local support that can facilitate any additional learning and other needs.

Relational Considerations

There are inherent challenges for supervisors in establishing and maintaining SRs using remote supervision, particularly if they have never met their supervisee in person. Supervisors and supervisees using telephone or online supervision do not have information available through non-verbal cues to inform and consolidate their relationship. Video-conferencing may provide some challenges in this area if there are interruptions due to problems with Internet connectivity. It may also be more difficult to be sensitive to unspoken relational issues or cultural differences.

Once again, the key to developing an effective SR in remote supervision is through careful, attentive contracting at the beginning of the relationship. The material discussed in Chapter 6 on contracting is relevant in this context. Additionally, the limitations and advantages of remote supervision can be made explicit and consideration given to how any limitations may be addressed. Careful consideration should be given to confidentiality and informed consent at the contracting phase. The use of a local back-up supervisor can be a helpful addition to remote supervision. This may be a useful adjunct and resource for the supervisee in case of an emergency but also for the supervisor if there are concerns about the supervisee's practice. This would need to be considered carefully with the supervisee at the contracting phase, and any decision to discuss issues of competence outside of the SR should be discussed in advance with the supervisee.

It is possible that the use of technology in supervision may heighten anxiety (Rousmaniere et al., 2014), and Rousmaniere and Ellis (2013) suggest that it is particularly important to emphasize collaboration in these supervisory relationships. Supervisors will need to work harder to tune in to their relationships with supervisees, to attend to verbal and (if possible) non-verbal cues. At the contracting phase of the relationship, supervisors should invite a discussion about the potential for misunderstanding or miscommunication that may be particularly relevant when using technology. Checking in and monitoring the relationship frequently, reviewing supervision regularly, and explicitly exploring the impact of the use of technology will also be important.

The use of technology in supervision offers many exciting possibilities for learning and enhancing practice. More research is needed into developing our understanding of the impact of technology on the SR, and into meeting the relational demands of supervision in this context.

Key Points

- Learning in groups can be a powerful experience, providing multiple opportunities for learning and normalizing anxieties, but it can provide a challenging interpersonal context if there are difficult group processes.
- Supervisors need knowledge and skills to manage group processes in addition to supervision skills
- Contracting is key, as are providing structure early on and clarity about the purpose, roles, and expectations of the group to promote a climate of cohesion and interpersonal trust.
- Making sense of problems should include consideration of group processes, contextual factors, and the contribution of individual supervisees and supervisor.
- The use of technology in supervision can provide significant opportunities for supervisee learning and development, and remote supervision can increase supervisory resource, particularly for those in remote areas.
- Confidentiality and informed consent are important ethical considerations when using technology.
- Contracting should invite discussion on the impact of technology and the potential for miscommunication.
- SRs should be monitored and reviewed regularly, and back-up arrangements should be specified if supervising remotely.

11

Summary and Conclusions

In summary, we believe that substantive conclusions can be drawn from the material that we have presented in this book. Supervision is central to, and the most significant aspect of, professional training in the majority of the helping professions across the world (Watkins & Milne, 2014). It is the contention of this book, which is well supported by the evidence, that the quality of the supervisory relationship is fundamental to both the experience of supervision and good supervision outcomes (Beinart & Clohessy, 2009). In this final chapter, we draw together findings from the literature and key practice issues to describe the features that are necessary for effective and competent SRs. Additionally, we provide some thoughts and guidance as to how supervisors and supervisees can effectively apply the material from this book in their day-to-day practice. Finally, we share some of our thoughts about the future of research and practice in this important and developing area.

Summary

Each chapter in this book describes a theme related to competent and effective SRs. The first five chapters in Part I focus on best evidence by reviewing and summarizing the academic literature. Chapter 1 outlines the significance of the SR in supervision research and practice, providing definitions of supervision and the SR, the influences of different contexts, and the importance of working within clear competency frameworks for supervision. Additionally, we describe in detail the work done in the UK clinical psychology training community by the Clinical Supervision Advisory Group (CSAG) on the 10 competencies required to develop effective supervisory relationships (Beinart & Golding, 2015).

Selected models of supervision, both those based on psychotherapy schools and those developed to explain the process of supervision itself, are discussed in Chapter 2. Other models that inform our understanding and practice of supervision are touched on, namely adult learning and attachment models. Models and frameworks of the SR are explored in some depth, including those developed by the Oxford Supervision Research Group, based on our qualitative research from the perspective of the supervisee (Beinart, 2014) and the supervisor (Clohessy, 2008).

Effective Supervisory Relationships: Best Evidence and Practice, First Edition.
Helen Beinart and Sue Clohessy.
© 2017 John Wiley & Sons Ltd. Published 2017 by John Wiley & Sons Ltd.

Chapter 3 describes the multiple influences on the SR, in particular supervisor, supervisee, dyadic, and contextual influences. The current evidence suggests that supervisors can create a safe space for learning by establishing clear boundaries and clarifying mutual expectations of the SR. Supervisors utilize therapeutic qualities such as active listening, empathy, respect, and acceptance to develop this safe space. Supervisors contribute by actively engaging with the supervisee. This involves being emotionally invested as well as available through a regular and predictable structure of supervision sessions. Additionally, supervisors encourage the supervisee to identify their learning needs, collaborate, and work together as a team. Supervisors can use appropriate self-disclosure to enhance the SR and to encourage supervisees to be honest and to share any issues that may be of concern. In addition to the supportive functions of supervision, supervisors also need to provide regular feedback and to initiate challenging discussions for effective SRs.

Supervisees contribute to effective SRs by remaining open to learning, receptive to feedback, and willing to consider and follow through supervision interventions. An enthusiastic, hardworking, and proactive stance contributes to an effective SR. Supervisees can also strengthen SRs by taking responsibility and appropriate autonomy for their work, and by being self-aware and able to reflect on and to critique their practice. Dyadic influences include the possible mirroring of the practice relationship within the SR; this is often referred to as parallel process. Additionally, attachment processes can influence the SR, in particular the supervisor's capacity to provide a safe base.

In Chapter 4 we discuss the outcome and measurement of SRs, and identify the key findings related to supervision outcomes. There is good evidence that effective supervision contributes to supervisee satisfaction, awareness, self-efficacy, and confidence. In other words, we can claim, with reasonable certainty, that supervisees benefit from supervision by reporting or demonstrating improvement in their knowledge, confidence, and skills. The gold standard outcome of client change or improvement consequent on the supervisory process and relationship has yet to be conclusively supported by empirical research, although studies are beginning to emerge. However, this is a challenging area to research in a meaningful way, and we need to begin to include measures of supervision and the SR into therapeutic and other practice outcome studies. Routine outcome measurement in practice that then feeds the results of client measures of change into the supervisory process is a promising new development. One contribution has been the development of some robust measures of the SR by the Oxford Supervision Research Group. These, together with alternative measures of the SR, can be selected for use in future outcome studies. The best evidence to date suggests that the SR is a significant mutative factor in the process and outcomes of supervision.

All the current competency frameworks for supervision include diversity-sensitive practice and cultural competence as core competencies for clinical supervision, and much of the research concludes that a safe SR is crucial for cultural conversations to take place. In Chapter 5 we introduced values-based practice and cultural humility as useful meta-concepts that underpin ethically sound and culturally sensitive SRs. Ethics within the SR is significant at a number of levels (e.g., competence, confidentiality, due process) but, most importantly, it supports familiarization with and socialization to the unique ethical stance of a particular profession. We see this ethical approach as intimately linked with diversity-sensitive practice through cultural curiosity and humility. Best evidence suggests that conversations about power and difference are more likely to take place in safe SRs where supervisees are supported to discuss and disclose their beliefs, values, and opinions.

Part II of this book focuses on best practice in the development and maintenance of effective SRs. The development of an agreement about mutual expectations and working practices through contracting is, in our view, the best way to start the SR. We see contracting (Chapter 6) as an initial mutual agreement that sets the tone for the relationship and requires ongoing review. Initial contracting begins a conversation, offers a model, and sets the agenda for what can be discussed in the future by raising potential issues that can be explored more fully as the relationship develops. In many ways, it is the genuineness of the real relationship, the process of the discussions, the openness and curiosity, rather than the content per se, that create the emotional climate for a collaborative and safe SR.

While effective contracting may be a way to get the SR off to a good start and to provide a solid foundation for the process, the giving and receiving of feedback (Chapter 7) can be seen as the fundamental work within supervision. Summative methods of feedback such as evaluation and assessment often dominate discussions of feedback. However, we have argued that formative feedback provided honestly and regularly throughout the SR is a core function of supervision and can often reduce the anxiety inherent in the process of giving and receiving summative feedback. Current best evidence suggests that supervisors do not provide enough detailed feedback to their supervisees. Methods to support effective feedback include effective goal-setting and contracting for feedback preferences, facilitating the process of constructive challenge, and self-assessment. We believe that regularly reviewing supervision and inviting supervisee feedback is a method of maintaining and strengthening the SR. Mutual feedback is integral to effective supervision and is most effective in the context of a safe and supportive SR.

Chapter 8 discusses managing difficulties within the SR. Some form of conflict is almost inevitable in SRs because of the tension between some of the functions of supervision, most notably the tension between the tasks of providing support and of evaluating or monitoring practice. Effective SRs are set up to minimize conflict by contracting carefully and by engaging in regular and honest mutual feedback. However, it is likely that there will be some strains and it is helpful for supervisors to adopt a stance of openness to conflict and to monitor the SR for signs of strain. A cycle of noticing, information-gathering, formulation, and intervention is a helpful way to approach tensions or strains in the SR. Current evidence suggests that approach and constructive challenging, rather than avoidance, is characteristic of effective SRs. We believe that the majority of practitioners do not use models of supervision sufficiently to help formulate and make sense of relationship strains or difficulties. This is an area where the use of a framework can depersonalize conflict and increase the likelihood of a positive resolution. Indeed, the successful management of difficulties is a valuable learning experience and may well strengthen the SR.

Reflective practice (Chapter 9) is another core function of supervision, and establishing optimal conditions for reflection is a key task within the SR. Studies of reflective practice suggest that a supportive learning environment, authenticity, and sensitivity to individual differences in learning styles and needs encourage reflection. There are numerous methods to facilitate reflective practice, including the use of contracting, questionnaires to explore learning preferences, and conversations about culture and difference. Additionally, creative methods, live supervision, the use of recording, and reflective writing are all helpful methods to encourage reflection within the SR. An important element of reflective practice is being self-aware and mindful of the impact we have on others. Part of the supervisory task is to facilitate this capacity in those whom we supervise. However, we are aware that many working environments are stressful and we include a section on self-care, noticing and managing stress, and building supervisory resources in order to facilitate resilience in both supervisors and supervisees.

In Chapter 10, we explore formats of supervision that go beyond the dyadic or one-to-one direct formats that were the focus of the preceding chapters. We discuss the theory and evidence relating to group supervision and the emerging material on the use of technology in the supervisory relationship, including through remote supervision. These alternative formats have become increasingly popular in recent years because of time pressures in many organizational settings, with group supervision now being the seen as a more economic or preferred option in some. Groups can be a very powerful context within which to learn, and the advantages of learning from each other through sharing multiple perspectives and normalizing the anxieties or other feelings that arise from the challenges of the work are significant. However, the relational tasks for the supervisor in group supervision are complex, requiring attention to group as well as supervisory processes. Supervisors need to create a safe and secure context to promote group cohesion. Using contracting, developing clear aims and ground rules for the group, and providing a clear structure early on are important ways to do this. If there are difficulties in the group, supervisors will need to consider multiple factors to make sense of these including, for example, the stage of group development, group processes, contextual influences on the group, as well as the individual contributions of supervisor and supervisees and the work that is being discussed.

The growth of technology has provided additional learning opportunities in the supervisory relationship, and, furthermore, it has created opportunities to provide supervision at a distance to those practicing in remote or rural settings who may previously have had limited access to supervision. These technological advances are exciting, providing opportunities for more in-depth and focused supervision on both supervisee and client outcomes (e.g., through the use of video-conferencing as a means of providing live supervision, or incorporating the data provided by client outcome software into the supervision agenda). Similarly, the opportunity to access supervision without the pragmatic boundaries of distance and geography through the use of technology is also a significant step forward. However, there are particular ethical issues to consider in supervisory relationships in these contexts, particularly relating to confidentiality and

Table 11.1 Characteristics of effective and competent supervisory relationships.

- Development of a supportive, collaborative, and open SR with clear boundaries to create a safe space that enables disclosure of any concerns.
- Active commitment to, and engagement with, supervision and the SR.
- Establishment of agreed, mutual goals, tasks, and expectations on the basis of individual learning needs and appropriate competency frameworks for supervision and practice.
- Application of models of supervision and the SR to aid the process of supervision and the use of these to understand and formulate or conceptualize any strains in the relationship.
- Keeping abreast of the research on supervisor, supervisee, dyadic, and contextual influences on the SR and applying these in practice.
- Use of a range of robust measures to monitor the diverse outcomes in supervision including supervisee, supervisor, and client perspectives.
- Employment of ethical and diversity- and/or culture-sensitive practice that values difference in all its forms and recognizes and manages power.
- Effective contracting for the SR, as well as for the nature of the supervision and the work to be supervised, and incorporation of a mechanism for regular review.
- Engagement of both parties in regular, balanced, and honest mutual feedback and challenge.
- Acknowledgement, prevention, and management of any strains or difficulties as soon as they arise.
- Utilization of reflective practice to explore the SR, supervision, and ongoing practice.
- Using reflective practice to monitor stress and to develop resources to ensure resilience in the workplace.

data security, informed consent, and due process (if there are concerns about supervisee competence). Supervisory relationships that are carried out at a distance do not have the benefit of supervisor and supervisee being able to get to know each through working together in a shared service setting, and may have to contend with technological problems that interfere with the flow of the supervision session. Contracting and review of the SR that explicitly cover these issues may be helpful. The impact of the use of technology in supervision is a growing area, and one that warrants further study.

Throughout this book, we have highlighted the key characteristics of effective supervisory relationships. Table 11.1 summarizes these central features, and the next section highlights the implications for practice and future directions.

Integration and Messages for Practice

For Supervisees

Supervisees have a significant role and multiple tasks in contributing to making supervision work effectively. Much of this work can be done by preparing well for each new SR and supervision session. This may include reflecting on their own needs and learning and feedback preferences, and arriving at each supervision session prepared with material that they wish to discuss. Good supervision is collaborative and requires both parties to invest in and to commit to making things work well. Supervisees may at times feel anxious or resistant and it is their responsibility to take ownership of these feelings and to spend some time reflecting on them. This may include reflecting on their background and influences, past experiences, and cultural contexts. It is important to consider whether any of their feelings and experiences are related to the SR, working context, or other issues. For example, a client may trigger resonances in their personal life that make them feel uncomfortable and this is an issue that should be raised in supervision to ensure best practice. Additionally, the supervisor may misinterpret the supervisee's discomfort (if this has not been shared) and this could impact the SR. However, the supervisee may need to consider how open they wish to be, so that they can moderate how much personal material they are comfortable in sharing without leaving themselves feeling vulnerable. Supervisees often experience normal concerns about competence or about whether they can trust their supervisor to respond sensitively to the issues that they choose to disclose. Often, these feelings are related to the asymmetrical power inherent within the SR.

Supervisees can actively engage with the SR and the working context by contributing to a genuine and open relationship, taking appropriate autonomy, and being clear about their needs and concerns. Additionally they can actively contribute to the SR by being curious, by showing enthusiasm for learning, and by a general commitment to the work. Supervisees have an important role in supporting and guiding the supervisory skills of their supervisor so that the supervision they receive is tailored to their particular needs. Effective SRs are shaped by the active engagement, behavior, and feedback provided by supervisees.

For Supervisors

It can feel overwhelming for supervisors to cover all the features identified in Table 11.1, and it can be challenging to know where to start. It may be that a supervisor already believes that their supervisory practice is good enough, and the long lists of competencies may make them feel anxious, overwhelmed, or resistant. A good place to start is with some of the exercises in Chapter 9. Reflecting on their practice will enable supervisors to work out what they are already doing well and the areas that could be worked on or improved. At the core of supervision is placing a high value on continuing to develop one's own practice and helping others to develop. However, this takes time and energy and these are often in short supply in busy working lives. We suggest that supervisors pick one area that they think they can improve on and work on one thing at a time. For example, if they think they could improve on contracting with supervisees, they can set some time aside in their supervision sessions to review the contract and check whether supervision is currently meeting their supervisees' needs. They could invite supervisees to give feedback and let them know that their views are valued and that they (the supervisor) wishes to work collaboratively with them. This sends a meta-message about how the supervisor wishes to work. Supervisors can keep a reflective log to help track their experiences and note any patterns that emerge. The evidence suggests that supervisees like more specific feedback, so supervisors could experiment with giving more feedback and note whether it impacts their SRs. If they are not comfortable with discussions of power or difference within their SRs, supervisors could use some of the exercises in Chapter 9 to explore their own cultural influences and invite their supervisees to do likewise. Many supervisors are uncomfortable with the inherent power vested in the SR. However, the power differential can be addressed by active collaboration and by supervisors facilitating the empowerment of supervisees. Finally, and perhaps most importantly, supervisors should step back and reflect on their supervisory practice, take any concerns to their own supervision, and consider further training in areas that they would like to change or develop.

For Supervisory Dyads

The SR is a unique relationship that requires careful balancing of multiple, often conflictual, tasks. For example, the relationship needs to balance both support and challenge, openness and keeping appropriate boundaries, instructing and encouraging autonomy, following agreed goals and supporting creativity, evaluating or monitoring performance and encouraging risk-taking, and so on. All of these tasks and functions sit in a creative tension with one another and the true craft of supervision is making informed judgements in the relational space between supervisor and supervisee about how, when, and how much to share, support, intervene, feedback, challenge, and take risks. There is genuinely no right way of doing this other than to acknowledge the complexity and multi-layered nature of the SR and be to open about the process. We believe that creating a meta-conversation, so that you can step back from the process of the SR, and have a conversation about it, is one way to approach this complexity. This involves both parties being curious and open in recognizing that it is their particular, unique SR that is theirs to shape, learn from, and enjoy.

For Organizations/Systems

Supervision is central to professional development and is essential for safe practice in organizations, helping staff to manage complex settings. There is some evidence to suggest that supervision can buffer the stresses of the job and increase resilience and staff well-being. It is key to clinical governance in organizations because it has both supportive and monitoring functions. Most of the helping professions learn their professional craft through supervision and it is required post-qualification in many professions. However, despite the evidence, some organizations do not prioritize or support supervision. This can be manifested in a lack of space or time allocated for staff to conduct supervision. An organizational ethos that overvalues client contact at the cost of supervision can result in supervisees experiencing supervision as yet another burden or demand in an already overstretched day or week. This should raise alarm bells because of the monitoring function of supervision and its contribution to safe practice. It is recommended that organizations have a supervision policy that requires all staff to receive a minimum of monthly supervision and to undergo training in supervision. The research suggests that monthly supervision is needed to develop a safe enough SR to address any issues that emerge. If supervision is conducted in groups, these should be small enough for safe SRs to develop. It is essential for supervisees to disclose mistakes or concerns. Supervision is likely to be the most appropriate space for supervisees to disclose and learn from mistakes, thereby supporting safe practice. Organizations would benefit from a systemic approach that incorporates and values supervision as part of its ethos and culture. This requires leaders who are knowledgeable about, committed to, and invested in the role that supervision plays in improving staff well-being and practice.

Future Directions

There is now substantive evidence on the qualities of effective SRs and on the multiple influences on the supervisory dyad. We have shared the evidence and our perspectives on the significant contribution that the SR makes to the process and outcome of supervision but we are still in the early stages of understanding the mechanisms of change. Contributions to early research into the SR were largely based on the supervisory working alliance and satisfaction with supervision because of the availability of sound measures of these constructs, and so there are few robust measures of the wider construct of the SR. However, the availability of the alliance and satisfaction measures has quite possibly narrowed the research findings and the theoretical understanding of the relationship between supervisor and supervisee. Indeed, Tangen and Borders (2016), in a recent conceptual review, stress the complexity and multi-layered nature of the SR and raise the difficulty various theorists have had in capturing all of its elements. We have made an attempt at this in our definition in Chapter 1. However, until we have some broad agreement on the conceptualization of the SR and the competencies involved, we are unlikely to be able to subject it to full and comprehensive study.

There are some interesting new ideas in the literature that we think have some parallels with our research and merit further investigation. Watkins and Milne (2014), in the conclusion of their book, raise the issue of the "real" relationship in supervision, that is, the personal rather than (or as well as) the professional relationship. This is a translational concept from psychotherapy research (Markin, Kivlighan, Gelso, Hummel, & Spiegel, 2014) that has yet to be specifically studied in supervision research. We feel that much of our work supports the idea of a "real" relationship. For example, in Clohessy's (2008) study, supervisors described spending more informal time together with their supervisees as a strategy for approaching strains in the SR. Being open and honest, and connecting and investing on an interpersonal and emotional level, would also suggest the existence and importance of a real or genuine relationship that is required for the development of a safe base. Understanding this "real" relationship can be complex. Rieck, Callahan, and Watkins (2015) have recently found that the variable of agreeableness in the supervisor's personality is inversely related to client outcomes in supervision. This is an interesting finding that suggests that an agreeable supervisor and a pleasant SR are not sufficient for effective supervision. This finding confirms anecdotal reports that supervisees need to be stretched and that too much comfort within the SR is not helpful. The task for supervisors, therefore, is to provide challenge as well as safety in their relationships with supervisees. A possible direction for future research is to explore the role of challenge within the SR.

Additionally, the findings from Rieck, Callahan, and Watkins (2015) provide some support for the framework and process of the SR based on the necessary and sufficient conditions for learning, proposed in Beinart's model of the SR (2012).

The development of a collaborative and safe relationship is necessary for supervision to take place effectively, while the educational, feedback, and monitoring tasks are also essential, although they are effective only in the context of a safe SR. Additionally, this study found a supervisee personality variable of "openness to experience," which is remarkably similar to the "openness to learning" construct in Clohessy's (2008) model. Taken together, these findings point to some promising new directions for research that go further than simply describing the characteristics of effective SRs, and begin to shed some light on some of the possible mechanisms within the relationship. There is an increasing trend in research to suggest that supervisors and supervisees report some similarities, but also some differences, in their experiences of the SR. When we set out to develop our measures, the intention was to find a single common measure of the SR for both supervisor and supervisee, but our findings have led us to a different understanding that reflects the different experiences and values of both supervisor and supervisee. The core relational variables that we have described as intrinsic to, and developing from, a safe base in our measures appear to be similar for supervisors and supervisees, but several studies suggest differences, including elements to do with evaluation, culture, power, challenge, mindfulness, and so on. We need further research to develop our conceptualization of the SR and to explore any further differences between supervisors and supervisees. Bernard and Goodyear (2014) suggest that the SR may be a mediating variable in all supervision research findings. Consequently, we need further research to explore how the SR mediates and interacts with other supervision outcomes such as client change and supervisee learning. Client change continues to be held up as the gold standard in outcome research in this field. However, until measurement of the SR becomes normative practice in client outcome studies, we are unlikely to be able to provide the evidence needed to support this standard. The development of robust measures of the SR will enable future studies to measure the supervisory relationship alongside other variables to distinguish its unique contribution. It would also be advantageous if, in the future, therapeutic and other practice outcome studies regularly incorporate measures of supervision and the SR to explore the multiple factors that may influence client change. We hold the view that the SR is crucial to other significant outcomes, namely, the effective learning and development of professional skills, confidence, and competence. Effective SRs provide the safe learning environment and experience needed to translate these significant professional competencies into practice settings. The SR is an important and influential relationship that can have a number of positive outcomes in addition to client change, including shaping the next generation of professionals (as in training SRs), facilitating others to develop their professional skills, and supporting them with the challenges of their work.

Endnote

We want to conclude this book with some reflections on our own SR, which at the time of writing has spanned 25 years and has seen many transitions. We met when SC was in her second year of training as a clinical psychologist, beginning a training placement with children and families, and HB was already an experienced supervisor and head of a child psychology service. Although HB was an experienced supervisor, like many practitioners, she was not fully aware of the literature on supervision at that time (the early 1990s), and largely used her own experience and supervisor role models to guide her supervision practice. As our initial SR was part of a training program, we would have contracted for the learning outcomes required, the goals and tasks of the supervisory working alliance (Bordin, 1983). It was so long ago that we cannot recall whether we had any formal negotiation and agreement specifically about the SR. However, many of the ingredients for a successful working relationship, and elements of what is now termed the "real relationship," were present. For example, SC remembers feeling apprehensive about working with children and families for the first time, and was able to be open and to disclose these anxieties. HB normalized this, and demonstrated that she was committed and invested in the relationship, by tuning into SC's identified learning needs and providing opportunities for SC to observe her work, offering a graded approach to working independently, as well as reassurance and constructive feedback, and building on SC's strengths. Although the SR was a boundaried relationship that focused on the development of SC's skills and the provision of a clinical service, both of us demonstrated an openness and willingness to be known as people (as well as professionals), which consolidated the growing trust and safety within the SR at this time. This was partly achieved by sharing our diverse personal histories and cultural backgrounds and the discovery that we had worked in the same geographical area in the past and shared some memories of previous supervisors and role models. This could be seen as the beginning of a cultural genogram that contributed to the development of the bond element of the working alliance (Bordin, 1983). Over time, our SR has had a number of role transitions. At the end of SC's training placement, HB was appointed to work on the training program where SC was training, and became her clinical tutor. This role involved organizing and monitoring the final year of SC's clinical training. Early on in this new role relationship, SC experienced a strain in another training SR and requested help in managing this.

Effective Supervisory Relationships: Best Evidence and Practice, First Edition.
Helen Beinart and Sue Clohessy.
© 2017 John Wiley & Sons Ltd. Published 2017 by John Wiley & Sons Ltd.

Their previous positive SR enabled SC to feel safe enough to disclose her concerns despite the fact that there was an evaluative element to HB's role on the training program. Once SC's training was completed, there was an interval in their relationship in which SC worked as a newly qualified clinical psychologist in an adult mental health setting, and HB continued working on the clinical psychology training program at the Oxford Institute of Clinical Psychology Training, eventually taking on the role of clinical and professional director. Once SC had been qualified for two years, HB encouraged her to consider supervising for the program. During this time, SC developed competence and confidence as a supervisor by providing clinical placements in adult mental health, as well as supervising other professionals in her team. HB was clinical tutor for one of these placements, this time supporting SC in a supervisor role for a trainee clinical psychologist. They continued to have intermittent contact whereby HB acted as a "distant presence" on the program, experienced by SC as a safe base. After several years, SC was appointed as a clinical tutor on the training program and HB once again became her supervisor, and her line manager (a new role), a phase of their relationship that lasted for 13 years until HB retired from her post. This phase involved managing the potential for ethical infringements involved in multiple relationships (clinical, managerial, and research supervision) and grappling with some of the issues inherent in wearing multiple metaphorical hats. During this time, HB encouraged SC's growing interest in the field of supervision, and they worked closely together in planning and delivering a range of trainings for supervisors. SC took the lead in developing a new introductory training course for supervisors and at this stage the SR became more equal and collaborative. HB also became SC's research supervisor for her doctoral research on the SR (Clohessy, 2008). As it was a piece of qualitative research, it was necessary to be reflexive about the influences of our SR on the research, a process that we both found challenging and interesting and that deepened both our SR and reflective practice skills. This phase of our relationship was characterized by collaboration and high levels of trust and mutual disclosure, an important mentoring aspect for SC. Feedback has felt unproblematic in the SR, perhaps because of the sense of openness, safety, and trust that continued to develop. Challenge has been welcomed and we have experienced supervision as a mutually enriching and valued space. In many ways, Holloway's (1995) model of the SR describes the relationship well. There has been negotiation of power and involvement over phases of the SR and, over time, a noticeable shift of power to a less hierarchical and more involved structure.

The most recent phase of our relationship has perhaps been the most challenging. Since HB retired, we no longer have a formal SR but continue to work together on a number of teaching and academic projects. This has included setting up a new Post-Graduate Certificate in Supervision aimed at a wide range of practitioners in health, education, business, and social care settings, and, of course, writing this book. SC is director of the supervision course and HB is a tutor so our relationship has evolved into one where SC has more hierarchical power. According to the French and Raven (1959) model, HB has lost her formal reward and coercive power but perhaps still holds some expert and referent power. However this is explained, the power in our relationship has shifted over time, as we have shared more responsibility and developed a more collaborative SR. We have often treated our SR with some degree of playfulness and lightness of touch, but this latest phase of our relationship has necessitated a willingness to "let go" (HB) and to "step up" (SC). Again, a foundation of safety and trust has enabled us to explore these issues. Our SR has endured a number of transitions of roles and responsibilities, in changing professional contexts (clinical services, training doctoral students, training supervisors) and changing family life span and personal circumstances. As may be expected over a quarter of a century, our working, personal, and family contexts have shifted significantly over time and there have been many challenges to negotiate along the way. In many ways we have personally grappled with many of the issues raised in this book. However, we believe that the early foundations, shared values, interests (particularly in supervision), the capacity to communicate, shift, be flexible, and adapt to changing circumstances, plus a fair dose of humor have all contributed to an effective and mutually beneficial SR.

Appendix 1

The Supervisory Relationship Questionnaire (SRQ)

Please tick the column which matches your opinion most closely.

The following statements describe some of the ways a person may feel about his/her supervisor. To what extent do you agree or disagree with each of the following statements about your relationship with your supervisor?	Strongly disagree	Disagree	Slightly disagree	Neither agree nor disagree	Slightly agree	Agree	Strongly agree
SAFE BASE SUBSCALE							
1. My supervisor was respectful of my views and ideas	1	2	3	4	5	6	7
2. My supervisor and I were equal partners in supervision	1	2	3	4	5	6	7
3. My supervisor had a collaborative approach in supervision	1	2	3	4	5	6	7
4. I felt safe in my supervision sessions	1	2	3	4	5	6	7
5. My supervisor was non-judgemental in supervision	1	2	3	4	5	6	7
6. My supervisor treated me with respect	1	2	3	4	5	6	7
7. My supervisor was open-minded in supervision	1	2	3	4	5	6	7
8. Feedback on my performance from my supervisor felt like criticism	7	6	5	4	3	2	1
9. The advice I received from my supervisor was prescriptive rather than collaborative	7	6	5	4	3	2	1

(*Continued*)

Effective Supervisory Relationships: Best Evidence and Practice, First Edition.
Helen Beinart and Sue Clohessy.
© 2017 John Wiley & Sons Ltd. Published 2017 by John Wiley & Sons Ltd.

(Continued)

Please tick the column which matches your opinion most closely.

The following statements describe some of the ways a person may feel about his/her supervisor. To what extent do you agree or disagree with each of the following statements about your relationship with your supervisor?	Strongly disagree	Disagree	Slightly disagree	Neither agree nor disagree	Slightly agree	Agree	Strongly agree
10. I felt able to discuss my concerns with my supervisor openly	1	2	3	4	5	6	7
11. Supervision felt like an exchange of ideas	1	2	3	4	5	6	7
12. My supervisor gave feedback in a way that felt safe	1	2	3	4	5	6	7
13. My supervisor treated me like an adult	1	2	3	4	5	6	7
14. I was able to be open with my supervisor	1	2	3	4	5	6	7
15. I felt that if I discussed my feelings openly with my supervisor I would be negatively evaluated	7	6	5	4	3	2	1

STRUCTURE SUBSCALE

16. My supervision sessions took place regularly	1	2	3	4	5	6	7
17. Supervision sessions were structured	1	2	3	4	5	6	7
18. My supervisor made sure that our supervision sessions were kept free from interruptions	1	2	3	4	5	6	7
19. Supervision sessions were regularly cut short by my supervisor	7	6	5	4	3	2	1
20. Supervision sessions were focused	1	2	3	4	5	6	7
21. My supervision sessions were disorganised	7	6	5	4	3	2	1
22. My supervision sessions were arranged in advance	1	2	3	4	5	6	7
23. My supervisor and I both drew up an agenda for supervision together	1	2	3	4	5	6	7

COMMITMENT SUBSCALE

24. My supervisor was enthusiastic about supervising me	1	2	3	4	5	6	7

Please tick the column which matches your opinion most closely.

The following statements describe some of the ways a person may feel about his/her supervisor. To what extent do you agree or disagree with each of the following statements about your relationship with your supervisor?	Strongly disagree	Disagree	Slightly disagree	Neither agree nor disagree	Slightly agree	Agree	Strongly agree
25. My supervisor appeared interested in supervising me	1	2	3	4	5	6	7
26. My supervisor appeared uninterested in me	7	6	5	4	3	2	1
27. My supervisor appeared interested in me as a person	1	2	3	4	5	6	7
28. My supervisor appeared to like supervising	1	2	3	4	5	6	7
29. I felt like a burden to my supervisor	7	6	5	4	3	2	1
30. My supervisor was approachable	1	2	3	4	5	6	7
31. My supervisor was available to me	1	2	3	4	5	6	7
32. My supervisor paid attention to my spoken feelings and anxieties	1	2	3	4	5	6	7
33. My supervisor appeared interested in my development as a professional	1	2	3	4	5	6	7
REFLECTIVE EDUCATION SUBSCALE							
34. My supervisor drew from a number of theoretical models	1	2	3	4	5	6	7
35. My supervisor drew from a number of theoretical models flexibly	1	2	3	4	5	6	7
36. My supervisor gave me the opportunity to learn about a range of models	1	2	3	4	5	6	7
37. My supervisor encouraged me to reflect on my practice	1	2	3	4	5	6	7
38. My supervisor linked theory and clinical practice well	1	2	3	4	5	6	7
39. My supervisor paid close attention to the process of supervision	1	2	3	4	5	6	7

(Continued)

(Continued)

Please tick the column which matches your opinion most closely.

The following statements describe some of the ways a person may feel about his/her supervisor. To what extent do you agree or disagree with each of the following statements about your relationship with your supervisor?	Strongly disagree	Disagree	Slightly disagree	Neither agree nor disagree	Slightly agree	Agree	Strongly agree
40. My supervisor acknowledged the power differential between supervisor and supervisee	1	2	3	4	5	6	7
41. My relationship with my supervisor allowed me to learn by experimenting with different therapeutic techniques	1	2	3	4	5	6	7
42. My supervisor paid attention to my unspoken feelings and anxieties	1	2	3	4	5	6	7
43. My supervisor facilitated interesting and informative discussions in supervision	1	2	3	4	5	6	7
44. I learnt a great deal from observing my supervisor	1	2	3	4	5	6	7

ROLE MODEL SUBSCALE

	Strongly disagree	Disagree	Slightly disagree	Neither agree nor disagree	Slightly agree	Agree	Strongly agree
45. My supervisor was knowledgeable	1	2	3	4	5	6	7
46. My supervisor was an experienced clinician	1	2	3	4	5	6	7
47. I respected my supervisor's skills	1	2	3	4	5	6	7
48. My supervisor was knowledgeable about the organizational system in which they worked	1	2	3	4	5	6	7
49. Colleagues appeared to respect my supervisor's views	1	2	3	4	5	6	7
50. I respected my supervisor as a professional	1	2	3	4	5	6	7
51. My supervisor gave me practical support	1	2	3	4	5	6	7
52. I respected my supervisor as a clinician	1	2	3	4	5	6	7

Please tick the column which matches your opinion most closely.

The following statements describe some of the ways a person may feel about his/her supervisor. To what extent do you agree or disagree with each of the following statements about your relationship with your supervisor?	Strongly disagree	Disagree	Slightly disagree	Neither agree nor disagree	Slightly agree	Agree	Strongly agree
53. My supervisor was respectful of clients	1	2	3	4	5	6	7
54. I respected my supervisor as a person	1	2	3	4	5	6	7
55. My supervisor appeared uninterested in his/her clients	7	6	5	4	3	2	1
56. My supervisor treated their colleagues with respect	1	2	3	4	5	6	7

FORMATIVE FEEDBACK SUBSCALE

57. My supervisor gave me helpful negative feedback on my performance	1	2	3	4	5	6	7
58. My supervisor was able to balance negative feedback on my performance with praise	1	2	3	4	5	6	7
59. My supervisor gave me positive feedback on my performance	1	2	3	4	5	6	7
60. My supervisor's feedback on my performance was constructive	1	2	3	4	5	6	7
61. My supervisor paid attention to my level of competence	1	2	3	4	5	6	7
62. My supervisor helped me identify my own learning needs	1	2	3	4	5	6	7
63. My supervisor did not consider the impact of my previous skills and experience on my learning needs	7	6	5	4	3	2	1
64. My supervisor thought about my training needs	1	2	3	4	5	6	7
65. My supervisor gave me regular feedback on my performance	1	2	3	4	5	6	7

(Continued)

(Continued)

Please tick the column which matches your opinion most closely.

The following statements describe some of the ways a person may feel about his/her supervisor. To what extent do you agree or disagree with each of the following statements about your relationship with your supervisor?	Strongly disagree	Disagree	Slightly disagree	Neither agree nor disagree	Slightly agree	Agree	Strongly agree
66. As my skills and confidence grew, my supervisor adapted supervision to take this into account	1	2	3	4	5	6	7
67. My supervisor tailored supervision to my level of competence	1	2	3	4	5	6	7

Scoring key: Scored 1 (Strongly disagree) to 7 (Strongly agree); reverse scoring: scored 7 (Strongly disagree) to 1 (Strongly agree)
Source: Palomo, Beinart, & Cooper, 2010.

Appendix 2

The Short Supervisory Relationship Questionnaire (S-SRQ)

Please tick the column that matches your opinion most closely.

The following statements describe some of the ways a person may feel about their supervisor. To what extent do you agree or disagree with each of the following statements about your relationship with your supervisor?	Strongly disagree	Disagree	Slightly disagree	Neither agree nor disagree	Slightly agree	Agree	Strongly agree
SAFE BASE SUBSCALE							
1. My supervisor was approachable							
2. My supervisor was respectful of my views and ideas							
3. My supervisor gave me feedback in a way that felt safe							
4. My supervisor was enthusiastic about supervising me							
5. I felt able to openly discuss my concerns with my supervisor							
6. My supervisor was non-judgemental in supervision							
7. My supervisor was open-minded in supervision							
8. My supervisor gave me positive feedback on my performance							

(*Continued*)

Effective Supervisory Relationships: Best Evidence and Practice, First Edition.
Helen Beinart and Sue Clohessy.
© 2017 John Wiley & Sons Ltd. Published 2017 by John Wiley & Sons Ltd.

(Continued)

Please tick the column that matches your opinion most closely.

The following statements describe some of the ways a person may feel about their supervisor. To what extent do you agree or disagree with each of the following statements about your relationship with your supervisor?	Strongly disagree	Disagree	Slightly disagree	Neither agree nor disagree	Slightly agree	Agree	Strongly agree
9. My supervisor had a collaborative approach in supervision							
REFLECTIVE EDUCATION SUBSCALE							
10. My supervisor encouraged me to reflect on my practice							
11. My supervisor paid attention to my unspoken feelings and anxieties							
12. My supervisor drew flexibly from a number of theoretical models							
13. My supervisor paid close attention to the process of supervision							
14. My supervisor helped me identify my own learning/ training needs							
STRUCTURE SUBSCALE							
15. Supervision sessions were focused							
16. Supervision sessions were structured							
17. My supervision sessions were disorganised							
18. My supervisor made sure that our supervision sessions were kept free from interruptions							

Scoring key: Items 1–16 and 18 scored 1 (Strongly disagree) to 7 (Strongly agree); item 17 scored 7 (Strongly disagree) to 1 (Strongly agree).

Source: Cliffe, Beinart, & Cooper, 2014.

Appendix 3

The Supervisory Relationship Measure (SRM)

Please tick the column that matches your opinion most closely.

The following statements describe some of the ways you may feel about your trainee and aspects of your supervisory relationship with them. To what extent do you agree or disagree with each of the following statements about your relationship with your trainee?	Strongly disagree	Moderately disagree	Slightly disagree	Neither agree nor disagree	Slightly agree	Moderately agree	Strongly agree
SAFE BASE SUBSCALE							
1. My trainee is open about any difficulties they are experiencing	1	2	3	4	5	6	7
2. My trainee is reflective in supervision	1	2	3	4	5	6	7
3. There is a good emotional atmosphere in supervision with my trainee	1	2	3	4	5	6	7
4. My trainee is open and honest in supervision	1	2	3	4	5	6	7
5. My trainee is willing to learn new things	1	2	3	4	5	6	7
6. My trainee is enthusiastic about being on placement with me	1	2	3	4	5	6	7
7. I like my trainee	1	2	3	4	5	6	7
8. My trainee is open to new experiences on placement	1	2	3	4	5	6	7
9. My trainee appears able to give me honest and open feedback	1	2	3	4	5	6	7

(Continued)

Effective Supervisory Relationships: Best Evidence and Practice, First Edition.
Helen Beinart and Sue Clohessy.
© 2017 John Wiley & Sons Ltd. Published 2017 by John Wiley & Sons Ltd.

(Continued)

Please tick the column that matches your opinion most closely.

The following statements describe some of the ways you may feel about your trainee and aspects of your supervisory relationship with them. To what extent do you agree or disagree with each of the following statements about your relationship with your trainee?	Strongly disagree	Moderately disagree	Slightly disagree	Neither agree nor disagree	Slightly agree	Moderately agree	Strongly agree
10. My trainee seems to like me	1	2	3	4	5	6	7
11. My trainee and I have a good professional relationship	1	2	3	4	5	6	7
12. Supervision provides a safe space for my trainee to learn	1	2	3	4	5	6	7
13. My trainee is open-minded and curious	1	2	3	4	5	6	7
14. My trainee's style and my own style interact well	1	2	3	4	5	6	7
15. My trainee values my experiences and skills	1	2	3	4	5	6	7

Safe Base Subscale Score =

SUPERVISOR COMMITMENT SUBSCALE

	Strongly disagree	Moderately disagree	Slightly disagree	Neither agree nor disagree	Slightly agree	Moderately agree	Strongly agree
16. I try to pitch things at the right level for my trainee	1	2	3	4	5	6	7
17. I keep my trainee's needs in mind	1	2	3	4	5	6	7
18. I try to ensure my trainee has adequate space and resources	1	2	3	4	5	6	7
19. I prepared for my trainee prior to their placement	1	2	3	4	5	6	7
20. I am available and accessible to my trainee	1	2	3	4	5	6	7
21. I look out for clinical work and other opportunities for my trainee	1	2	3	4	5	6	7
22. I attempt to facilitate reflection in supervision with my trainee	1	2	3	4	5	6	7
23. I set up regular supervision for my trainee	1	2	3	4	5	6	7
24. I give clear and honest feedback to my trainee	1	2	3	4	5	6	7

Supervisor Commitment Subscale Score =

Please tick the column that matches your opinion most closely.

The following statements describe some of the ways you may feel about your trainee and aspects of your supervisory relationship with them. To what extent do you agree or disagree with each of the following statements about your relationship with your trainee?	Strongly disagree	Moderately disagree	Slightly disagree	Neither agree nor disagree	Slightly agree	Moderately agree	Strongly agree
TRAINEE CONTRIBUTION SUBSCALE							
25. My trainee is able to hold an appropriate case load	1	2	3	4	5	6	7
26. My trainee appears to be doing the minimum required	7	6	5	4	3	2	1
27. My trainee works hard on placement	1	2	3	4	5	6	7
28. My trainee copes well with multiple demands	1	2	3	4	5	6	7
29. My trainee is considerate toward others in the service (e.g., secretaries)	1	2	3	4	5	6	7
30. My trainee shows good organizational skills	1	2	3	4	5	6	7
31. My trainee shows poor professional values	7	6	5	4	3	2	1
32. My trainee takes appropriate responsibility for their work	1	2	3	4	5	6	7
33. My trainee behaves appropriately in the team	1	2	3	4	5	6	7
34. My trainee produces good-quality work	1	2	3	4	5	6	7
35. My trainee integrates well with others in the team	1	2	3	4	5	6	7
36. I am disappointed by my trainee's level of skill	7	6	5	4	3	2	1
37. I value having my trainee on placement	1	2	3	4	5	6	7
Trainee Contribution Subscale Score =							
EXTERNAL INFLUENCES SUBSCALE							
38. My trainee tries to use supervision as therapy	7	6	5	4	3	2	1

(*Continued*)

(Continued)

Please tick the column that matches your opinion most closely.

The following statements describe some of the ways you may feel about your trainee and aspects of your supervisory relationship with them. To what extent do you agree or disagree with each of the following statements about your relationship with your trainee?	Strongly disagree	Moderately disagree	Slightly disagree	Neither agree nor disagree	Slightly agree	Moderately agree	Strongly agree
39. My trainee's past experiences of supervision interfere with our relationship	7	6	5	4	3	2	1
40. My trainee has other life stressors which distract them from their work	7	6	5	4	3	2	1
41. Things to do with the trainee's course interfere with placement	7	6	5	4	3	2	1
42. I have stressors in my life which make it difficult for me to focus on supervision	7	6	5	4	3	2	1
43. I sense that my trainee worries because I am evaluating them	7	6	5	4	3	2	1
44. Evaluation has a negative impact on our relationship	7	6	5	4	3	2	1
45. My trainee is too anxious to engage in supervision	7	6	5	4	3	2	1

External Influences Subscale Score =

SUPERVISOR INVESTMENT SUBSCALE

46. I am aware of what interests my trainee	1	2	3	4	5	6	7
47. I am open in my supervision with my trainee	1	2	3	4	5	6	7
48. I try to get to know my trainee	1	2	3	4	5	6	7
49. I am able to share my strengths and my weaknesses with my trainee	1	2	3	4	5	6	7
50. Supervision is a safe place for me to give negative feedback	1	2	3	4	5	6	7

Please tick the column that matches your opinion most closely.

The following statements describe some of the ways you may feel about your trainee and aspects of your supervisory relationship with them. To what extent do you agree or disagree with each of the following statements about your relationship with your trainee?	Strongly disagree	Moderately disagree	Slightly disagree	Neither agree nor disagree	Slightly agree	Moderately agree	Strongly agree
51. I have a good idea about what my trainee wants to gain from this placement	1	2	3	4	5	6	7

Supervisor Investment Subscale Score =

SRM TOTAL SCORE =

Scoring instructions: Subscale scores = Sum of individual item scores within the subscale. The mean item score is calculated by dividing the sum by the number of items in the subscale. Total SRM score = Sum of five subscale scores. The mean item score is calculated by dividing the total by 51.

Note: Items 26, 31, 36, 38, 39, 40, 41, 42, 43, 44, and 45 are reverse-scored and the item scores have already been adjusted in the above measure.

Source: Pearce, Beinart, Clohessy, & Cooper, 2013.

References

Abbass, A., Arthey, S., Elliott, J., Fedak, T., Nowoweiski, D., Markovski, J., & Nowoweiski, S. (2011). Web-conference supervision for advanced psychotherapy training: A practical guide. *Psychotherapy, 48*(2), 109–118.

Allen, G. J., Szollos, S. J., & Williams, B. E. (1986). Doctoral students' comparative evaluations of best and worst psychotherapy supervision. *Professional Psychology: Research and Practice, 17*(2), 91–99. doi: 10.1037/0735-7028.17.2.91

Alonso, A., & Rutan, J. S. (1988). Shame and guilt in psychotherapy supervision. *Psychotherapy: Theory, Research, Practice, Training, 25*(4), 576–581.

American Psychological Association. (2015). Guidelines for clinical supervision in health service psychology. *The American Psychologist, 70*(1), 33–46.

Amundson, N. E. (1988). The use of metaphor and drawings in case conceptualization. *Journal of Counseling & Development, 66*(8), 391–393.

Andersen, T. (1987). The reflecting team: Dialogue and meta-dialogue in clinical work. *Family Process, 26*(4), 415–428.

Anderson, S. A., Schlossberg, M., & Rigazio-DiGilio, S. (2000). Family therapy trainees' evaluations of their best and worst supervision experiences. *Journal of Marital and Family Therapy, 26*(1), 79–91.

Argyris, C., & Schon, D. A. (1974). *Theory in practice: Increasing professional effectiveness*. San Francisco: Jossey-Bass.

Bahrick, A. S. (1990). Role induction for counselor trainees: Effects on the supervisory working alliance. Ohio State University. *Dissertation Abstracts International, 51*, 1484B. (University Microfilms No. 90-14, 392)

Bakker, A. B., Demerouti, E., & Euwema, M. C. (2005). Job resources buffer the impact of job demands on burnout. *Journal of Occupational Health Psychology, 10*(2), 170–180.

Bambling, M. (2000). The effect of clinical supervision on the development of counsellor competency. *Psychotherapy in Australia, 6*(4), 58–63.

Bambling, M. (2014). Creating positive outcomes in clinical supervision. In C. E. Watkins & D. L. Milne (Eds.), *The Wiley International Handbook of Clinical Supervision* (pp. 445–457). Chichester, UK: Wiley Blackwell.

Bambling, M., & King, R. (2014). Supervisor social skill and supervision outcome. *Counselling and Psychotherapy Research, 14*(4), 256–262.

Effective Supervisory Relationships: Best Evidence and Practice, First Edition.
Helen Beinart and Sue Clohessy.
© 2017 John Wiley & Sons Ltd. Published 2017 by John Wiley & Sons Ltd.

Bambling, M., King, R., Raue, P., Schweitzer, R., & Lambert, W. (2006). Clinical supervision: Its influence on client-rated working alliance and client symptom reduction in the brief treatment of major depression. *Psychotherapy Research, 16*(3), 317–331.

Bandura, A. (1986). *Social foundations of thought and action: A social cognitive theory*. Englewood Cliffs, NJ: Prentice Hall.

Barnes, K. L. (2004). Applying self-efficacy theory to counselor training and supervision: A comparison of two approaches. *Counselor Education and Supervision, 44*(1), 56–69.

Barrett-Lennard, G. T. (1962). Dimensions of therapist response as causal factors in therapeutic change. *Psychological Monographs: General and Applied, 76*(43), 1–36.

Beauchamp, T. L., & Childress, J. F. (1994). *Principles of medical ethics*. Oxford: Oxford University Press.

Beauchamp, T. L., & Childress, J. F. (2013). *Principles of medical ethics* (7th ed.). Oxford: Oxford University Press.

Beck, A. T., Rush, A. J., Shaw, B. F., & Emery, G. (1979). *Cognitive therapy of depression*. New York: Guilford Press.

Beinart, H. (2002). *An exploration of the factors which predict the quality of the relationship in clinical supervision*. Unpublished DClinPsych thesis, Open University, UK.

Beinart, H. (2012). Models of supervision and the supervisory relationship. In I. Fleming & L. Steen (Eds.), *Supervision and clinical psychology: Theory, practice and perspectives* (pp. 36–50). Hove, UK, and New York : Brunner-Routledge.

Beinart, H. (2014). Building and sustaining the supervisory relationship. In C. E. Watkins & D. L. Milne (Eds.), *The Wiley International Handbook of Clinical Supervision* (pp. 255–281). Chichester, UK: Wiley Blackwell.

Beinart, H., & Clohessy, S. (2009). Supervision. In H. Beinart, P. Kennedy, & S. Llewelyn (Eds.), *Clinical Psychology in Practice* (pp. 319–335). Oxford: Wiley Blackwell.

Beinart, H., & Clohessy, S. (2016). Clinical supervision. In N. Tarrier & J. Johnson (Eds.), *Case Formulation in Cognitive Behaviour Therapy* (pp. 352–369). London: Routledge.

Beinart, H., & Golding, L. (2015). Group of Trainers in Clinical Psychology Training and Recognition (STAR) guidance on learning outcomes for advanced supervisor training: The desired characteristics of experienced and effective clinical psychology supervisors. *Clinical Psychology Forum, 266*, 30–35.

Bennett, C. S. (2008). Attachment-informed supervision for social work field education. *Clinical Social Work Journal, 36*(1), 97–107.

Bennett, S., & Deal, K. H. (2009). Beginnings and endings in social work supervision: The interaction between attachment and developmental processes. *Journal of Teaching in Social Work, 29*(1), 101–117.

Bennett, S., Mohr, J., BrintzenhofeSzoc, K., & Saks, L. V. (2008). General and supervision-specific attachment styles: Relations to student perceptions of field supervisors. *Journal of Social Work Education, 44*(2), 75–94.

Bennett, S., & Saks, L. V. (2006). Field notes: A conceptual application of attachment theory and research to the social work student–field instructor supervisory relationship. *Journal of Social Work Education, 42*(3), 669–682.

Bennett-Levy, J. (2006). Therapist skills: A cognitive model of their acquisition and refinement. *Behavioural and Cognitive Psychotherapy, 34*, 57–78.

Bennett-Levy, J., & Lee, N. K. (2014). Self-practice and self-reflection in cognitive behaviour therapy training: What factors influence trainees' engagement and experience of benefit? *Behavioural and Cognitive Psychotherapy, 42*, 48–64. doi: 10.1017/S1352465812000781

Bennett-Levy, J., Thwaites, R., Haarhoff, B., & Perry, H. (2015). *Experiencing CBT from the Inside Out: A Self-Practice/Self-Reflection Workbook for Therapists.* New York: Guilford Press.

Bernard, J. M. (1979). Supervisor training: A discrimination model. *Counselor Education and Supervision, 19*(1), 60–68.

Bernard, J. M. (1997). The discrimination model. In C. E. Watkins (Ed.), *Handbook of Psychotherapy Supervision* (pp. 310–327). New York: Wiley.

Bernard, J. M., & Goodyear, R. (2014). *Fundamentals of Clinical Supervision* (5th ed.). Harlow, UK: Pearson.

Blackburn, I.-M., James, I. A., Milne, D. L., Baker, C., Standart, S., Garland, A., & Reichelt, F. K. (2001). The revised cognitive therapy scale (CTS-R): Psychometric properties. *Behavioural and Cognitive Psychotherapy, 29*(4), 431–446.

Boëthius, S. B., & Ögren, M. L. (2000). Role patterns in group supervision. *The Clinical Supervisor, 19*, 45–69.

Boëthius, S. B., Sundin, E., & Ögren, M. L. (2006). Group supervision from a small group perspective. *Nordic Psychology, 58*(1), 22–42.

Borders, L. D. (1991). Developmental changes during their supervisees' first practicum. *The Clinical Supervisor, 8*(2), 157–167.

Bordin, E. S. (1979). The generalizability of the psychoanalytic concept of the working alliance. *Psychotherapy: Theory, Research & Practice, 16*(3), 252–260.

Bordin, E. S. (1983). Supervision in counseling II. Contemporary models of supervision: A working alliance based model of supervision. *The Counseling Psychologist, 11*(1), 35–42.

Borsay, C. (2012). *Understanding the supervisory relationship and what happens when difficulties occur.* Unpublished DClinPsych thesis, University of Oxford.

Bradshaw, T., Butterworth, A., & Mairs, H. (2007). Does structured clinical supervision during psychosocial intervention education enhance outcome for mental health nurses and the service users they work with? *Journal of Psychiatric and Mental Health Nursing, 14*(1), 4–12.

British Psychological Society. (2009). *Code of ethics and conduct.* Leicester: BPS.

Brown, B., & Marzillier, J. S. (1993). *The evaluation of clinical competence.* Report on the proceedings of the Joint CUCPT and CORIC workshop held at Grasmere, Cumbria, UK.

Burkard, A. W., Knox, S., Clarke, R. D., Phelps, D. L., & Inman, A. G. (2014). Supervisors' experiences of providing difficult feedback in cross-ethnic/racial supervision. *The Counseling Psychologist, 42*(3), 314–344.

Burkard, A. W., Knox, S., Hess, S. A., & Schultz, J. (2009). Lesbian, gay, and bisexual supervisees' experiences of LGB-affirmative and nonaffirmative supervision. *Journal of Counseling Psychology, 56*(1), 176–188.

Burnham, J. (2005). Systemic supervision: The evolution of reflexivity in the context of the supervisory relationship. *Human Systems, 4*, 349–381.

Burnham, J. (2010). Creating reflexive relationships between practices of systemic supervision and theories of learning and education. In C. Burck & G. Daniel (Eds.), *Mirrors and reflections: Processes of systemic supervision* (pp. 49–78). London: Karnac.

Burnham, J. (2011). Developments in Social GRRRAAACCEEESSS: Visible–invisible and voiced–unvoiced. In I.-B. Krause (Ed.), *Culture and reflexivity in systemic psychotherapy: Mutual perspectives* (pp. 139–160). London: Karnac.

Burnham, J., Alvis Palma, D., & Whitehouse, L. (2008). Learning as a context for differences and differences as a context for learning. *Journal of Family Therapy, 30*(4), 529–542.

Burnham, J., & Harris, Q. (2002). Cultural issues in supervision. In D. Campbell & B. Mason (Eds.), *Perspectives on Supervision* (pp. 21–41). London: Karnac

Callahan, J. L., Almstrom, C. M., Swift, J. K., Borja, S. E., & Heath C. J. (2009). Exploring the contribution of supervisors to intervention outcomes. *Training and Education in Professional Psychology, 3*(2), 72–77.

Carey, J. C., Williams, K. S., & Wells, M. (1988). Relationships between dimensions of supervisors' influence and counselor trainees' performance. *Counselor Education and Supervision, 28*(2), 130–139.

Carifio, M. S., & Hess, A. K. (1987). Who is the ideal supervisor? *Professional Psychology: Research and Practice, 18*(3), 244–250. doi: 10.1037/0735-7028.18.3.244

Carlson, L., Rapp, C. A., & Eichler, M. S. (2012). The experts rate: Supervisory behaviors that impact the implementation of evidence-based practices. *Community Mental Health Journal, 48*(2), 179–186.

Carroll, M. (1996). *Counseling supervision: Theory, skills and practice.* London: Cassell.

Carroll, M., & Gilbert, M. (2005). *On being a supervisor: Creating learning partnerships.* London: Vukani.

Cashwell, T. H., & Dooley, K. (2001). The impact of supervision on counselor self-efficacy. *The Clinical Supervisor, 20*(1), 39–47.

Cassidy, S. (2004). Learning styles: An overview of theories, models, and measures. *Educational Psychology, 24*(4), 419–444.

Celano, M. P., Smith, C. O., & Kaslow, N. J. (2010). A competency-based approach to couple and family therapy supervision. *Psychotherapy: Theory, Research, Practice, Training, 47*(1), 35–44.

Cherniss, C., & Egnatios, E. (1977). Styles of clinical supervision in community mental health programs. *Journal of Consulting and Clinical Psychology, 45*(6), 1195–1196.

Cliffe, T., Beinart, H., & Cooper, M. (2014). Development and validation of a short version of the Supervisory Relationship Questionnaire. *Clinical Psychology & Psychotherapy, 23*(1), 77–86.

Clohessy, S. (2008). *Supervisors' perspectives on their supervisory relationships: A qualitative study.* Unpublished PsyD thesis, University of Hull, UK.

Clynes, M. (2004). *An exploratory study of preceptors' views and experiences of providing feedback on clinical performance to post-registration student nurses (sick children's nursing).* Unpublished master's thesis, University of Dublin, Ireland.

Clynes, M. P., & Raftery, S. E. (2008). Feedback: An essential element of student learning in clinical practice. *Nurse Education in Practice, 8*(6), 405–411.

Cobia, D. C., & Boes, S. R. (2000). Professional disclosure statements and formal plans for supervision: Two strategies for minimizing the risk of ethical conflicts in post-master's supervision. *Journal of Counseling & Development, 78*(3), 293–296.

Conn, J. J. (2002). What can clinical teachers learn from *Harry Potter and the Philosopher's Stone*? *Medical Education, 36*(12), 1176–1181.

Cooper, L., & Gustafson, J. P. (1985). Supervision in a group: An application of group theory. *The Clinical Supervisor, 3*(2), 7–25.

Corrie, S., & Lane, D. A. (2015). *CBT Supervision*. London: SAGE.

Crockett, S., & Hays, D. G. (2015). The influence of supervisor multicultural competence on the supervisory working alliance, supervisee counseling self-efficacy, and supervisee satisfaction with supervision: A mediation model. *Counselor Education and Supervision, 54*, 258–273. doi: 10.1002/ceas.12025

Cummings, P. (2002). Cybervision: Virtual peer group counselling supervision— Hindrance or help? *Counselling and Psychotheraphy Research, 2*(4), 223–229.

Cushway, D., & Tyler, P. A. (1994). Stress and coping in clinical psychologists. *Stress Medicine, 10*(1), 35–42.

Daniel, L., Borders, L. D., & Willse, J. (2015). The role of supervisors' and supervisees' mindfulness in clinical supervision. *Counselor Education and Supervision, 54*, 221–232.

Deal, K. H., Bennett, S., Mohr, J., & Hwang, J. (2011). Effects of field instructor training on student competencies and the supervisory alliance. *Research on Social Work Practice, 21*(6), 712–726.

De Luque, M. F. S., & Sommer, S. M. (2000). The impact of culture on feedback-seeking behavior: An integrated model and propositions. *Academy of Management Review, 25*(4), 829–849.

Dewey, J. (1933). *How we think*. Buffalo, NY: Prometheus.

Dickson, J. M., Moberly, N. J., Marshall, Y., & Reilly, J. (2011). Attachment style and its relationship to working alliance in the supervision of British clinical psychology trainees. *Clinical Psychology & Psychotherapy, 18*(4), 322–330.

Division of Clinical Psychology, British Psychological Society. (2014). *DCP Policy on Supervision*. Leicester, UK: BPS.

Dohrenwend, A. (2002). Serving up the feedback sandwich. *Family Practice Management, 9*(10), 43–50.

Doughty, E. A., & Leddick, G. R. (2007). Gender differences in the supervisory relationship. *Journal of Professional Counseling Practice Theory and Research, 35*(2), 17–30.

Dye, H. A., & Borders, L. D. (2011). Counseling supervisors : Standards for preparation and practice. *Journal of Counseling and Development, 69*(1), 27–29. doi: 10.1002/j.1556-6676.1990.tb0149

Efstation, J. F., Patton, M. J., & Kardash, C. M. (1990). Measuring the working alliance in counselor supervision. *Journal of Counseling Psychology, 37*(3), 322–329.

Ekstein, R., & Wallerstein, R. S. (1972). *The teaching and learning of psychotherapy* (revised ed.). Oxford: International Universities Press.

Ellis, M. V. (2010). Bridging the science and practice of clinical supervision: Some discoveries, some misconceptions. *The Clinical Supervisor, 29*(1), 95–116.

Ellis, M. V., Berger, L., Hanus, A. E., Ayala, E. E., Swords, B. A., & Siembor, M. (2014). Inadequate and harmful clinical supervision testing a revised framework and assessing occurrence. *The Counseling Psychologist, 42*(4), 434–472.

Ellis, M. V., D'Iuso, N., & Ladany, N. (2008). State of the art in the assessment, measurement, and evaluation of clinical supervision. *Psychotherapy Supervision: Theory, Research, and Practice, 2,* 473–499.

Ellis, M. V., & Douce, L. A. (1994). Group supervision of novice clinical supervisors: Eight recurring issues. *Journal of Counseling and Development, 72*(5), 520–525.

Ellis, M. V., & Ladany, N. (1997). Inferences concerning supervisees and clients in clinical supervision: An integrative review. In C. E. Watkins (Ed.), *Handbook of psychotherapy supervision* (pp. 447–507). Hoboken, NJ: Wiley.

Elman, N. S., & Forrest, L. (2007). From trainee impairment to professional competence problems: Seeking new terminology that facilitates effective action. *Professional Psychology: Research and Practice, 38*(5), 501–509.

Falender, C. A. (2014a). Supervision outcomes: Beginning the journey beyond the emperor's new clothes. *Training and Education in Professional Psychology, 8*(3), 143–148.

Falender, C. A. (Ed.). (2014b). Supervision outcomes [Special issue]. *Training and Education in Professional Psychology, 8*(3).

Falender, C. A., Burnes, T. R., & Ellis, M. V. (2013). Multicultural clinical supervision and benchmarks empirical support informing practice and supervisor training. *The Counseling Psychologist, 41*(1), 8–27.

Falender, C. A., Collins, C. J., & Shafranske, E. P. (2009). "Impairment" and performance issues in clinical supervision: After the 2008 ADA Amendments Act. *Training and Education in Professional Psychology, 3*(4), 240–249.

Falender, C. A., & Shafranske, E. P. (2004). *Clinical supervision: A competency approach.* Washington, DC : American Psychological Association.

Falender, C. A., & Shafranske, E. P. (2007). Competence in competency-based supervision practice: Construct and application. *Professional Psychology: Research and Practice, 38*(3), 232–240.

Falender, C. A., & Shafranske, E. P. (2012). *Getting the most out of clinical training and supervision: A guide for practicum students and interns.* Washington, DC: American Psychological Association.

Falender, C. A., & Shafranske, E. P. (2014). Clinical supervision: State of the art. *Journal of Clinical Psychology, 70*(11), 130–141. doi: xs10.1002/jclp

Falender, C. A., Shafranske, E. P., & Falicov, C. J. (2014). *Multiculturalism and diversity in clinical supervision: A competency-based approach.* Washington, DC: American Psychological Association.

Farber, B. A. (2006). Supervisee and supervisor disclosure. In B. A. Farber, *Self Disclosure in Psychotherapy* (pp. 180–197). New York: Guilford Press.

Farber, E. W. (2012). Supervising humanistic-existential psychotherapy: Needs, possibilities. *Journal of Contemporary Psychotherapy, 42*(3), 173–182.

Farber, E. W. (2014). Supervising humanistic and existential psychotherapies. In C. E. Watkins & D. L. Milne (Eds.) *The Wiley International Handbook of Clinical Supervision* (pp 530–551). Chichester : Wiley Blackwell.

Farmer, S. S. (1987). Conflict management and clinical supervision. *The Clinical Supervisor, 5*(3), 5–28.

Fleming, I., & Steen, L. (2013). *Supervision and clinical psychology: Theory, practice and perspectives.* London: Routledge.

Fleming, L. M., Glass, J. A., Fujisaki, S., & Toner, S. L. (2010). Group process and learning: A grounded theory model of group supervision. *Training and Education in Professional Psychology, 4*(3), 194–203.

Foster, J. T., Lichtenberg, J. W., & Peyton, V. (2007). The supervisory attachment relationship as a predictor of the professional development of the supervisee. *Psychotherapy Research, 17*(3), 343–350.

Frawley-O'Dea, M. G. (2003). Supervision is a relationship too: A contemporary approach to psychoanalytic supervision. *Psychoanalytic Dialogues, 13*(3), 355–366.

Frawley-O'Dea, M. G., & Sarnat, J. E. (2001). *The supervisory relationship: A contemporary psychodynamic approach.* New York: Guilford Press.

Freitas, G. J. (2002). The impact of psychotherapy supervision on client outcome: A critical examination of 2 decades of research. *Psychotherapy: Theory, Research, Practice, Training, 39*(4), 354–367.

French, J. and Raven, B. (1959). The bases of social power. In D. Cartwright (Ed.), *Studies in social power* (pp. 150–167). Ann Arbor, MI: Institute for Social Research.

Fulford, K. (2008). Values-based practice: A new partner to evidence-based practice and a first for psychiatry? *Mens Sana Monographs, 6*(1), 10–21.

Gatmon, D., Jackson, D., Koshkarian, L., Martos-Perry, N., Molina, A., Patel, N., & Rodolfa, E. (2001). Exploring ethnic, gender, and sexual orientation variables in supervision: Do they really matter? *Journal of Multicultural Counseling and Development, 29*(2), 102–113.

Gauthier, J. (2008). The Universal Declaration of Ethical Principles for Psychologists. In J. E. Hall & E. M. Altmaier (Eds.), *Global Promise: Quality Assurance and Accountability in Professional Psychology* (pp. 98–108). New York: Oxford University Press.

Gauthier, J., & Pettifor, J. (2012). The tale of two universal declarations: Ethics and human rights. In M. M. Leach, M. J. Stevens, G. Lindsay, A. Ferrero, & Y. Korkut (Eds.), *The Oxford Handbook of International Psychological Ethics* (pp. 113–133). Oxford: Oxford University Press.

Gilfoyle, N. (2008). The legal exosystem: Risk management in addressing student competence problems in professional psychology training. *Training and Education in Professional Psychology, 2*(4), 202–209.

Gonsalvez, C. J. (2014). Establishing supervision goals and formalizing a supervision agreement. In C. E. Watkins & D. L. Milne (Eds.), *The Wiley International Handbook of Clinical Supervision* (pp. 282–307). Chichester, UK: Wiley Blackwell.

Granello, D. H., Beamish, P. M., & Davis, T. E. (1997). Supervisee empowerment: Does gender make a difference? *Counselor Education and Supervision, 36*(4), 305–317.

Grant, J., Schofield, M. J., & Crawford, S. (2012). Managing difficulties in supervision: supervisors' perspectives. *Journal of Counseling Psychology, 59*(4), 528–541.

Gray, L. A., Ladany, N., Walker, J. A., & Ancis, J. R. (2001). Psychotherapy trainees' experience of counterproductive events in supervision. *Journal of Counseling Psychology, 48*(4), 371–383.

Green, D. R. (1998). *Investigating the core skills of clinical supervision: A qualitative analysis.* Unpublished DClinPsych thesis, University of Leeds, UK.

Grossl, A. B., Reese, R. J., Norsworthy, L. A., & Hopkins, N. B. (2014). Client feedback data in supervision: Effects on supervision and outcome. *Training and Education in Professional Psychology, 8*, 182–188.

Guest, C. L., & Dooley, K. (1999). Supervisor malpractice: Liability to the supervisee in clinical supervision. *Counselor Education and Supervision, 38*(4), 269–279.

Guiffrida, D. A., Jordan, R., Saiz, S., & Barnes, K. L. (2007). The use of metaphor in clinical supervision. *Journal of Counseling & Development, 85*(4), 393–400.

Hannigan, B., Edwards, D., & Burnard, P. (2004). Stress and stress management in clinical psychology: Findings from a systematic review. *Journal of Mental Health, 13*(3), 235–245.

Hansen, N. D., Randazzo, K. V., Schwartz, A., Marshall, M., Kalis, D., Frazier, R., & Norvig, G. (2006). Do we practice what we preach? An exploratory survey of multicultural psychotherapy competencies. *Professional Psychology: Research and Practice, 37*(1), 66–74.

Harbin, J. J., Leach, M. M., & Eells, G. T. (2008). Homonegativism and sexual orientation matching in counseling supervision. *Counselling Psychology Quarterly, 21*(1), 61–73.

Hattie, J., & Timperley, H. (2007). The power of feedback. *Review of Educational Research, 77*(1), 81–112.

Hawkins, P., & Shohet, R. (2006). *Supervision in the helping professions.* Berkshire, England: Open University Press.

Hawkins, P., & Shohet, R. (2012). *Supervision in the helping professions.* Maidenhead, UK: Open University Press.

Heckman-Stone, C. (2004). Trainee preferences for feedback and evaluation in clinical supervision. *The Clinical Supervisor, 22*(1), 21–33.

Heid, L. (1998). Supervisor development across the professional lifespan. *The Clinical Supervisor, 16*, 139–152.

Henderson, C. E., Cawyer, C. S., & Watkins, C. E. (1999). A comparison of student and supervisor perceptions of effective practicum supervision. *The Clinical Supervisor, 18*(1), 47–74. doi: 10.1300/J001v18n01_04

Hess, A. K., Hess, K. D., & Hess, T. H. (2008). *Psychotherapy supervision: Theory, research, and practice.* Hoboken, NJ: Wiley.

Hess, S. A., Knox, S., Schultz, J. M., Hill, C. E., Sloan, L., Brandt, S., & Hoffman, M. A. (2008). Predoctoral interns' nondisclosure in supervision. *Psychotherapy Research, 18*(4), 400–411.

Hill, C., & Knox, S. (2013). Training and supervision in psychotherapy. In M. J. Lambert (Ed.), *Bergin and Garfield's Handbook of Psychotherapy and Behavior Change* (pp. 775–811). Hoboken, NJ: Wiley.

Hoffman, M. A., Hill, C. E., Holmes, S. E., & Freitas, G. F. (2005). Supervisor perspective on the process and outcome of giving easy, difficult, or no feedback to supervisees. *Journal of Counseling Psychology, 52*(1), 3–13.

Holloway, E. L. (1982). Interactional structure of the supervision interview. *Journal of Counseling Psychology, 29*(3), 309–317.

Holloway, E. L. (1995). *Clinical supervision: A systems approach.* Thousand Oaks, CA: SAGE.

Holloway, E. L. (2014). Supervisory roles within systems of practice. In C. E. Watkins & D. L. Milne (Eds.), *The Wiley International Handbook of Clinical Supervision* (pp. 598–621). Chichester, UK: Wiley Blackwell.

Holloway, E. L., & Poulin, K. L. (1995). Discourse in supervision. In S. Jurg (Ed.), *Therapeutic and everyday discourse as behaviour change: Towards a micro analysis in psychotherapy process research* (pp. 245–273). Westport, CT: Ablex.

Honey, P., & Mumford, A. (1992). *The manual of learning styles.* Maidenhead, UK: Peter Honey.

Howard, F. (2008). Managing stress or enhancing wellbeing? Positive psychology's contributions to clinical supervision. *Australian Psychologist, 43*(2), 105–113.

Howell, W. (1982). *The empathic communicator.* Wadsworth, CA: Belmont.

Hsu, W. (2009). The components of solution-focused supervision. *Bulletin of Educational Psychology, 41*(2), 475–496.

Hughes, J. (2012). Practical aspects of supervision: All you ever wanted to know but were too afraid to ask. In I. Fleming & L. Steen (Eds.), *Supervision and clinical psychology: Theory, practice and perspectives* (pp. 184–206). Hove, UK: Routledge.

Hutt, C. H., Scott, J., & King, M. (1983). A phenomenological study of supervisees' positive and negative experiences in supervision. *Psychotherapy: Theory, Research & Practice, 20*(1), 118–123.

Inman, A. G., Hutman, H., Pendse, A., Devdas, L., Luu, L., & Ellis, M. V. (2014). Current trends concerning supervisors, supervisees, and clients in clinical supervision. In C.E. Watkins & D.L Milne (Eds.), *The Wiley International Handbook of Clinical Supervision* (pp. 61–102). Chichester, UK: Wiley Blackwell.

Inman, A. G., & Ladany, N. (2008). Research: The state of the field. *Psychotherapy Supervision: Theory, Research, and Practice, 2,* 500–517.

Inman, A. G., Schlosser, L. Z., Ladany, N., Howard, E. E., Boyd, D. L., Altman, A. N., & Stein, E. P. (2011). Advisee nondisclosures in doctoral-level advising relationships. *Training and Education in Professional Psychology, 5*(3), 149–159.

Inskipp, F., & Proctor, B. (1993). *Making the most of supervision.* Twickenham, UK: Cascade.

Inskipp, F., & Proctor, B. (1995). *The art, craft and tasks of counseling supervision: Part 2. Becoming a supervisor.* Twickenham, UK: Cascade.

Ishiyama, F. (1988). A model of visual case processing using metaphors and drawings. *Counselor Education and Supervision, 28*(2), 153–161.

Jacobsen, C. H. (2007). A qualitative single case study of parallel processes. *Counselling & Psychotherapy Research, 7*(1), 26–33.

James, I. A. (2015). The rightful demise of the sh*t sandwich: Providing effective feedback. *Behavioural and Cognitive Psychotherapies, 43*(6), 759–766.

James, I. A., Milne, D., Marie-Blackburn, I., & Armstrong, P. (2007). Conducting successful supervision: Novel elements towards an integrative approach. *Behavioural and Cognitive Psychotherapy, 35*(2), 191–200.

Jernigan, M. M., Green, C. E., Helms, J. E., Perez-Gualdron, L., & Henze, K. (2010). An examination of people of color supervision dyads: Racial identity matters as much as race. *Training and Education in Professional Psychology, 4*(1), 62–73.

Jerome, P. J. (1994). *Coaching through effective feedback: A practical guide to successful communication.* London: Kogan Page.

Johnston, L. H., & Milne, D. L. (2012). How do supervisees learn during supervision? A grounded theory study of the perceived developmental process. *The Cognitive Behaviour Therapist, 5*(1), 1–23.

Kagan, N. (1984). Interpersonal process recall: Basic methods and recent research. In D. Larson (Ed.), *Teaching psychological skills* (pp. 229–244). Monterey, CA: Brooks/Cole.

Katzow, A. W., & Safran, J. D. (2007). Recognizing and resolving ruptures in the therapeutic alliance. In P. Gilbert & R. Leahy (Eds.), *The therapeutic relationship in the cognitive behavioral psychotherapies* (pp. 90–105). Hove, UK : Routledge.

Kauderer, S., & Herron, W. G. (1990). The supervisory relationship in psychotherapy over time. *Psychological Reports, 67*(2), 471–480.

Kavanagh, D. J., Spence, S. H., Strong, J., Wilson, J., Sturk, H., & Crow, N. (2003). Supervision practices in allied mental health: Relationships of supervision characteristics to perceived impact and job satisfaction. *Mental Health Services Research, 5*(4), 187–195.

Kennerley, H., & Clohessy, S. (2010). Becoming a supervisor. In M. Mueller, H. Kennerley, F. McManus, & D. Westbrook (Eds.), *Oxford Guide to Surviving as a CBT Therapist* (pp. 323–370). Oxford: Oxford University Press.

Knox, S., Edwards, L. M., Hess, S. A., & Hill, C. E. (2011). Supervisor self-disclosure: Supervisees' experiences and perspectives. *Psychotherapy, 48*(4), 336–341.

Koh, L. C. (2008). Refocusing formative feedback to enhance learning in pre-registration nurse education. *Nurse Education in Practice, 8*(4), 223–230.

Kolb, D. A. (1976). Management and the learning process. *California Management Review, 18*(3), 21–31.

Kolb, D. A. (1984). *Experiential learning: Experience as the source of learning and development.* Upper Saddle River, NJ: Prentice Hall.

Kolb, D. A. (2015). *Experiential learning: Experience as the source of learning and development* (2nd ed.). Upper Saddle River, NJ: Pearson Education.

Koltz, R. L., Odegard, M. A., Feit, S. S., Provost, K., & Smith, T. (2012). Parallel process and isomorphism: A model for decision making in the supervisory triad. *The Family Journal, 20*(3), 233–238.

Kozlowska, K., Nunn, K., & Cousens, P. (1997a). Training in psychiatry: An examination of trainee perceptions. Part 1. *Australian and New Zealand Journal of Psychiatry, 31*(5), 628–640.

Kozlowska, K., Nunn, K., & Cousens, P. (1997b). Adverse experiences in psychiatric training, Part 2. *Australian and New Zealand Journal of Psychiatry, 31*(5), 641–652.

Krause, I.-B. (1998). *Therapy across culture: Perspectives on psychotherapy.* Thousand Oaks, CA: SAGE.

Ladany, N. (2014). The ingredients of supervisor failure. *Journal of Clinical Psychology, 70*(11), 1094–1103.

Ladany, N., Constantine, M. G., Miller, K., Erickson, C. D., & Muse-Burke, J. L. (2000). Supervisor countertransference: A qualitative investigation into its identification and description. *Journal of Counseling Psychology, 47*(1), 102–115.

Ladany, N., Ellis, M. V. & Friedlander, M. L. (1999). The supervisory working alliance, trainee self-efficacy and satisfaction. *Journal of Counseling and Development, 77*, 447–455.

Ladany, N., & Friedlander, M. L. (1995). The relationship between the supervisory working alliance and trainees' experience of role conflict and role ambiguity. *Counselor Education and Supervision, 34*(3), 220–231.

Ladany, N., Friedlander, M. L., & Nelson, M. L. (2005). *Critical events in psychotherapy supervision: An interpersonal approach.* Washington, DC: American Psychological Association.

Ladany, N., Hill, C. E., Corbett, M. M., & Nutt, E. A. (1996). Nature, extent, and importance of what psychotherapy trainees do not disclose to their supervisors. *Journal of Counseling Psychology, 43*(1), 10–24.

Ladany, N., & Inman, A. (2008). Developments in counseling skills training and supervision. In S. D. Brown and R. W. Lent (Eds.), *Handbook of counseling psychology* (4th revised ed.) (pp. 338–354). Hoboken, NJ: Wiley.

Ladany, N., & Lehrman-Waterman, D. E. (1999). The content and frequency of supervisor self-disclosures and their relationship to supervisor style and the supervisory working alliance. *Counselor Education and Supervision, 38*(3), 143–160.

Ladany, N., & Melincoff, D. S. (1999). The nature of counselor supervisor nondisclosure. *Counselor Education and Supervision, 38*(3), 161–176.

Ladany, N., Mori, Y., & Mehr, K. W. (2013). Effective and ineffective supervision. *The Counseling Psychologist, 41*, 28–47.

Ladany, N., Walker, J., Pate-Carolan, L., & Evans, L. G. (2008). *Experiencing counselling and psychotherapy: Insights from psychotherapy trainees, their clients, and their supervisors.* New York: Taylor & Francis.

Lahad, M. (2000). *Creative supervision: The use of expressive arts methods in supervision and self-supervision.* London: Jessica Kingsley.

Leary, T. F. (1957). *Interpersonal diagnosis of personality: A functional theory and methodology for personality evaluation.* Oxford: Ronald Press.

Lehrman-Waterman, D., & Ladany, N. (2001). Development and validation of the evaluation process within supervision inventory. *Journal of Counseling Psychology, 48*(2), 168–177.

Lemoir, V. (2013). *Difference and disclosure in supervision.* Unpublished DClinPsych thesis, University of Oxford.

Liese, B. S., & Beck, J. S. (1997). Cognitive therapy supervision. In C. E. Watkins, Jr. (Ed.), *Handbook of Psychotherapy Supervision* (pp. 114–133). Hoboken, NJ : Wiley.

Loganbill, C., Hardy, E., & Delworth, U. (1982). Supervision: A conceptual model. *The Counseling Psychologist, 10*(1), 3–42.

Magnuson, S., Wilcoxon, S. A., & Norem, K. (2000). A profile of lousy supervision: Experienced counselors' perspectives. *Counselor Education and Supervision, 39*(3), 189–202.

Mann, K., Gordon, J., & MacLeod, A. (2009). Reflection and reflective practice in health professions education: a systematic review. *Advances in Health Sciences Education, 14*(4), 595–621.

Mannix, K. A., Blackburn, I. M., Garland, A., Gracie, J., Moorey, S., Reid, B., & Scott, J. (2006). Effectiveness of brief training in cognitive behaviour therapy techniques for palliative care practitioners. *Palliative Medicine, 20*(6), 579–584.

Markin, R. D., Kivlighan, D. M., Jr., Gelso, C. J., Hummel, A. M., & Spiegel, E. B. (2014). Clients' and therapists' real relationship and session quality in brief therapy: An actor partner interdependence analysis. *Psychotherapy, 51*(3), 413–423.

Mastoras, S. M., & Andrews, J. J. (2011). The supervisee experience of group supervision: Implications for research and practice. *Training and Education in Professional Psychology, 5*(2), 102–111.

Mayseless, O. (2010). Attachment and the leader–follower relationship. *Journal of Social and Personal Relationships, 27*(2), 271–280.

McCarthy, P., Kulakowski, D., & Kenfield, J. A. (1994). Clinical supervision practices of licensed psychologists. *Professional Psychology: Research and Practice, 25*(2), 177–181.

Mehr, K. E., Ladany, N., & Caskie, G. I. (2010). Trainee nondisclosure in supervision: What are they not telling you? *Counselling and Psychotherapy Research, 10*(2), 103–113.

Messinger, L. (2007). Supervision of lesbian, gay, and bisexual social work students by heterosexual field instructors: A qualitative dyad analysis. *The Clinical Supervisior, 26*(1–2), 195–222.

Milne, D. (2007). An empirical definition of clinical supervision. *British Journal of Clinical Psychology, 46*(4), 437–447.

Milne, D. (2009). *Evidence-based clinical supervision.* Chichester, UK: British Psychological Society/Blackwell.

Milne, D. L. (2014). Toward an Evidence-Based Approach to Clinical Supervision. In C. E. Watkins & D. L. Milne (Eds.), *The Wiley International Handbook of Clinical Supervision* (pp. 38–60). Chichester, UK: Wiley Blackwell.

Milne, D., & James, I. (2000). A systematic review of effective cognitive-behavioural supervision. *British Journal of Clinical Psychology, 39*(2), 111–127.

Milne, D. L., Kennedy, E., Todd, H. Lombardo, C., Freeston, M. & Day, A. (2008). Zooming in on clinical supervision. *Behavioural and Cognitive Psychotherapy, 36*, 619–624.

Milne, D., & Reiser, R. P. (2012). A rationale for evidence-based clinical supervision. *Journal of Contemporary Psychotherapy, 42*(3), 139–149.

Milne, D. L., & Watkins, C. E. (2014). Defining and understanding clinical supervision: A functional approach. In C. E. Watkins, & D. L. Milne (Eds.), *The Wiley International Handbook of Clinical Supervision* (pp. 3–19). Chichester, UK: Wiley Blackwell.

Moskowitz, S. A., & Rupert, P. A. (1983). Conflict resolution within the supervisory relationship. *Professional Psychology: Research and Practice, 14*(5), 632–641.

Mueller, W. J., & Kell, B. L. (1972). *Coping with conflict: Supervising counselors and psychotherapists.* East Norwalk, CT : Appleton-Century-Crofts.

Munson, C. (2012). *Handbook of Clinical Social Work Supervision.* New York: Haworth Social Work Practice.

Myrick, F., & Yonge, O. (2002). Preceptor behaviors integral to the promotion of student critical thinking. *Journal for Nurses in Professional Development, 18*(3), 127–133.

Narvaez, D., & Lapsley, D. K. (2005). The psychological foundations of everyday morality and moral expertise. *Character psychology and character education* (pp. 140–165). Notre Dame, IN: Notre Dame Press.

Nelson, G. L. (1978). Psychotherapy supervision from the trainee's point of view: A survey of preferences. *Professional Psychology, 9*(4), 539–550. doi: 10.1037/0735-7028.9.4.539

Nelson, M. L., Barnes, K. L., Evans, A. L., & Triggiano, P. J. (2008). Working with conflict in clinical supervision: Wise supervisors' perspectives. *Journal of Counseling Psychology, 55*(2), 172–184.

Nelson, M. L., & Friedlander, M. L. (2001). A close look at conflictual supervisory relationships: The trainee's perspective. *Journal of Counseling Psychology, 48*(4), 384–395.

Nelson, M. L., & Holloway, E. L. (1990). Relation of gender to power and involvement in supervision. *Journal of Counseling Psychology, 37*(4), 473–481.

Nerdrum, P., & Rønnestad, M. H. (2002). The Trainees' Perspective: A Qualitative Study of Learning Empathic Communication in Norway. *The Counseling Psychologist, 30*(4), 609–629. doi: 10.1177/00100002030004007

Neswald-McCalip, R. (2001). Development of the secure counselor: Case examples supporting Pistole & Watkins's (1995) discussion of attachment theory in counseling supervision. *Counselor Education and Supervision, 41*(1), 18–27.

Newman, C. F. (2010). Competency in conducting cognitive-behavioral therapy: Foundational, functional, and supervisory aspects. *Psychotherapy: Theory, Research, Practice, Training, 47*(1), 12–19.

Ng, K.-M., & Smith, S. D. (2012). Training level, acculturation, role ambiguity, and multicultural discussions in training and supervising international counseling students in the United States. *International Journal for the Advancement of Counselling, 34*(1), 72–86.

Norem, K., Magnuson, S., Wilcoxon, S. A., & Arbel, O. (2006). Supervisees' contributions to stellar supervision outcomes. *Journal of Professional Counselling, Practice & Theory, 34*(1–2), 33–48.

O'Donovan, A., & Kavanagh, D. J. (2014). Measuring competence in supervisees and supervisors. In C. E. Watkins & D. L. Milne (Eds.), *The Wiley International Handbook of Clinical Supervision* (pp. 458–467). Chichester, UK: Wiley Blackwell.

Ögren, M. L., Apelman, A., & Klawitter, M. (2001) The group in psychotherapy supervision. *The Clinical Supervisor, 20*(2), 147–176.

Ögren, M. L., Boëthius, S. B., & Sundin, E. (2014). Challenges and possibilities in group supervision. In E. Watkins & D. L. Milne (Eds.), *The Wiley International Handbook of Clinical Supervision* (pp. 648–669). Chichester, UK: Wiley Blackwell.

Ögren, M. L., & Sundin, E. C. (2007). Experiences of the group format in psychotherapy supervision. *The Clinical Supervisor, 25*(1–2), 69–82.

Olds, K., & Hawkins, R. (2014). Precursors to measuring outcomes in clinical supervision: A thematic analysis. *Training and Education in Professional Psychology, 8*(3), 158–164.

Olk, M. E., & Friedlander, M. L. (1992). Trainees' experiences of role conflict and role ambiguity in supervisory relationships. *Journal of Counseling Psychology, 39*(3), 389–397.

Osborn, C. J., & Davis, T. E. (1996). The supervision contract: Making it perfectly clear. *The Clinical Supervisor, 14*(2), 121–134.

Padesky, C. A. (1996). Developing cognitive therapist competency: Teaching and supervision models. In P. Salkovskis (Ed.), *Frontiers of Cognitive Therapy* (pp. 266–292). New York: Guilford Press.

Pakdaman, S., Shafranske, E., & Falender, C. (2014). Ethics in supervision: Consideration of the supervisory alliance and countertransference management of psychology doctoral students. *Ethics & Behavior, 25*(5), 427–441.

Palomo, M. (2004). *Development and validation of a questionnaire measure of the supervisory relationship (SRQ).* Unpublished DClinPsych thesis, University of Oxford.

Palomo, M., Beinart, H., & Cooper, M. J. (2010). Development and validation of the Supervisory Relationship Questionnaire (SRQ) in UK trainee clinical psychologists. *British Journal of Clinical Psychology, 49*(2), 131–149.

Panos, P. T. (2005). A model for using videoconferencing technology to support international social work field practicum students. *International Social Work, 48*(6), 834–841.

Patton, M. J., & Kivlighan, D. M., Jr. (1997). Relevance of the supervisory alliance to the counseling alliance and to treatment adherence in counselor training. *Journal of Counseling Psychology, 44*(1), 108–115.

Pearce, N., Beinart, H., Clohessy, S., & Cooper, M. (2013). Development and validation of the supervisory relationship measure: A self-report questionnaire for use with supervisors. *British Journal of Clinical Psychology, 52*(3), 249–268.

Pendleton, D., Schofield, T., Tate, P., & Havelock, P. (1984). *The consultation: An approach to teaching and learning.* Oxford: Oxford University Press.

Pettifor, J., McCarron, M. C., Schoepp, G., Stark, C., & Stewart, D. (2011). Ethical supervision in teaching, research, practice, and administration. *Canadian Psychology, 52*(3), 198–205.

Pettifor, J. L., & Sawchuk, T. R. (2006). Psychologists' perceptions of ethically troubling incidents across international borders. *International Journal of Psychology, 41*(3), 216–225.

Pettifor, J., Sinclair, C., & Falender, C. A. (2014). Ethical supervision: Harmonizing rules and ideals in a globalizing world. *Training and Education in Professional Psychology, 8*(4), 201–210.

Pistole, M. C., & Fitch, J. C. (2008). Attachment theory in supervision: A critical incident experience. *Counselor Education and Supervision, 47*(3), 193–205.

Pistole, M. C., & Watkins, C. E. (1995). Attachment theory, counselling process and supervision. *The Counseling Psychologist, 23*(3), 457–478.

Prieto, L. R. (1996). Group supervision: Still widely practiced but poorly understood. *Counselor Education and Supervision, 35*(4), 295–307.

Proctor, B., & Inskipp, F. (1988). Skills for supervising and being supervised. *St Leonards-on-Sea*, UK: Alexia.

Proctor, B., & Inskipp, F. (2001). Group supervision. In J. Scaife, *Supervision in the Helping Professions* (pp. 99–121). Hove, UK: Brunner-Routledge.

Proctor, B., & Inskipp, F. (2009). Group supervision. In J. Scaife, *Supervision in Clinical Practice* (2nd ed.) (pp. 137–163). London: Routledge.

Psychology Board of Australia. (2013). Guidelines for supervisors and supervisor training providers. Retrieved from http://www.psychologyboard.gov.au/ standards-and-guidelines/codes-guidelines-policies.aspx

Rabinowitz, F. E., Heppner, P. P., & Roehlke, H. J. (1986). Descriptive study of process and outcome variables of supervision over time. *Journal of Counseling Psychology, 33*(3), 292.

Raichelson, S. H., Herron, W. G., Primavera, L. H., & Ramirez, S. M. (1997). Incidence and effects of parallel process in psychotherapy supervision. *The Clinical Supervisor, 15*(2), 37–48.

Rakovshik, S. G., & McManus, F. (2013). An anatomy of CBT training: trainees' endorsements of elements, sources and modalities of learning during a postgraduate CBT training course. *The Cognitive Behaviour Therapist, 6*, e11. doi: 10.1017/S1754470X13000160

Ramos-Sánchez, L., Esnil, E., Goodwin, A., Riggs, S., Touster, L. O., Wright, L. K., & Rodolfa, E. (2002). Negative supervisory events: Effects on supervision and supervisory alliance. *Professional Psychology: Research and Practice, 33*(2), 197–202.

Reese, R. J., Usher, E. L., Bowman, D. C., Norsworthy, L. A., Halstead, J. L., Rowlands, S. R., & Chisholm, R. R. (2009). Using client feedback in psychotherapy training: An analysis of its influence on supervision and counselor self-efficacy. *Training and Education in Professional Psychology, 3*(3), 157–168.

Reichelt, S., Gullestad, S. E., Hansen, B. R., Rønnestad, M. H., Torgersen, A. M., Jacobsen, C. H., & Skjerve, J. (2009). Nondisclosure in psychotherapy group supervision: The supervisee perspective. *Nordic Psychology, 61*(4), 5–27.

Reiser, R. P., & Milne, D. (2012). Supervising cognitive-behavioral psychotherapy: Pressing needs, impressing possibilities. *Journal of Contemporary Psychotherapy, 42*(3), 161–171.

Renfro-Michel, E. L., & Sheperis, C. J. (2009). The relationship between counseling supervisee attachment orientation and perceived bond with supervisor. *The Clinical Supervisor, 28*(2), 141–154.

Richards, D. A. (2014). Clinical case management supervision. In C. E. Watkins & D. L. Milne (Eds.), *The Wiley International Handbook of Clinical Supervision* (pp. 518–529). Chichester, UK: Wiley Blackwell.

Rieck, T., Callahan, J. L., & Watkins, C. E., Jr. (2015). Clinical supervision: An exploration of possible mechanisms of action. *Training and Education in Professional Psychology, 9*(2), 187–194.

Rigazio-DiGilio, S. (2014). Common themes across systemic integrative supervision models. In T. C. Todd & C. L. Storm (Eds.), *The complete systemic supervisor: Context, philosophy, and pragmatics* (pp. 231–254). Chichester, UK: Wiley.

Riggs, S. A., & Bretz, K. M. (2006). Attachment processes in the supervisory relationship: An exploratory investigation. *Professional Psychology: Research and Practice, 37*(5), 558–566.

Robiner, W., Fuhrman, M., & Ristvedt, S. (1993). Evaluation difficulties in supervising psychology interns. *The Clinical Psychologist, 46*(1), 3–13.

Rodolfa, E., Bent, R., Eisman, E., Nelson, P., Rehm, L., & Ritchie, P. (2005). A cube model for competency development: implications for psychology educators and regulators. *Professional Psychology: Research and Practice, 36*(4), 347–354.

Rodolfa, E., Hall, T., Holms, V., Davena, A., Komatz, D., Antunez, M., & Hall, A. (1994). The management of sexual feelings in therapy. *Professional Psychology: Research and Practice, 25*(2), 168–172.

Rogers, C. R. (1957). The necessary and sufficient conditions of therapeutic personality change. *Journal of Consulting Psychology, 21*(2), 95–103.

Rønnestad, M. H., & Lundquist, K. (2009). The Brief Supervisory Alliance Scale—Trainee Form. Unpublished manuscript.

Rønnestad, M. H., & Skovholt, T. M. (2003). The journey of the counselor and therapist: Research findings and perspectives on professional development. *Journal of Career Development, 30*(1), 5–44.

Roth, A. D., & Pilling, S. (2007). *The competences required to deliver effective cognitive and behavioural therapy for people with depression and with anxiety disorders.* Retrieved from http://webarchive.nationalarchives.gov. uk/20130107105354/http://www.dh.gov.uk/en/Publicationsandstatistics/ Publications/PublicationsPolicyAndGuidance/DH_078537

Roth, A. D., & Pilling, S. (2008). Using an evidence-based methodology to identify the competences required to deliver effective cognitive and behavioural therapy for depression and anxiety disorders. *Behavioural and Cognitive Psychotherapy, 36*(2), 129–147.

Roth, A. D., Pilling, S., & Turner, J. (2010). Therapist training and supervision in clinical trials: Implications for clinical practice. *Behavioural and cognitive psychotherapy, 38*(3), 291–302.

Rousmaniere, T. G. (2014). Using technology to enhance clinical supervision and training. In C. E. Watkins & D. L. Milne (Eds.), *The Wiley International Handbook of Clinical Supervision* (pp. 204–237). Chichester, UK: Wiley Blackwell.

Rousmaniere, T., Abbass, A., & Frederickson, J. (2014). New developments in technology-assisted supervision and training: A practical overview. *Journal of Clinical Psychology, 70*(11), 1082–1093.

Rousmaniere, T. G., & Ellis, M. V. (2013). Developing the construct and measure of collaborative clinical supervision: The supervisee's perspective. *Training and Education in Professional Psychology, 7*(4), 300–308.

Rousmaniere, T., & Frederickson, J. (2013). Internet-based one-way-mirror supervision for advanced psychotherapy training. *The Clinical Supervisor, 32*(1), 40–55.

Rousseau, D. (1995). *Psychological contracts in organizations: Understanding written and unwritten agreements.* Thousand Oaks, CA: SAGE.

Safran, J. D., & Muran, J. C. (2001). A relational approach to training and supervision in cognitive psychotherapy. *Journal of Cognitive Psychotherapy, 15*(1), 3–15.

Sarnat, J. E. (2010). Key competencies of the psychodynamic psychotherapist and how to teach them in supervision. *Psychotherapy: Theory, Research, Practice, Training, 47*(1), 20–27.

Sarnat, J. E. (2012). Supervising psychoanalytic psychotherapy: Present knowledge, pressing needs, future possibilities. *Journal of Contemporary Psychotherapy, 42*(3), 151–160.

Satterly, B. A., & Dyson, D. (2008). Sexual minority supervision. *The Clinical Supervisor, 27*(1), 17–38.

Scaife, J. (2001). *Supervision in the mental health professions: A practitioner's guide.* London: Brunner-Routledge.

Scaife, J. (2009). *Supervision in Clinical Practice: A practitioner's guide.* London: Routledge.

Scaife, J. (2010). *Supervising the reflective practitioner: A essential guide to theory and practice.* London: Routledge.

Scaife, J., & Scaife, J. (2001). Supervision and learning. In J. Scaife, *Supervision in the mental health professions: A practitioner's guide* (pp. 15–29). Hove, UK: Brunner-Routledge.

Schacht, A. J., Howe, H. E., & Berman, J. J. (1989). Supervisor facilitative conditions and effectiveness as perceived by thinking- and feeling-type supervisees. *Psychotherapy: Theory, Research, Practice, Training, 26,* 475–483.

Schon, D. A. (1983). *The reflective practitioner.* New York: Basic Books.

Schon, D. A. (1987). *Educating the reflective practitioner.* San Francisco: Jossey-Bass.

Schütz, A. (1967). *The phenomenology of the social world.* Evanston, IL: Northwestern University Press.

Scott, T. L., Pachana, N. A., & Sofronoff, K. (2011). Survey of current curriculum practices within Australian postgraduate clinical training programmes: Students' and programme directors' perspectives. *Australian Psychologist, 46*(2), 77–89.

Sells, J. N. (1993). *The relationship between supervisor and trainee gender and their interactional behavior.* Doctoral dissertation, University of Southern California. *Dissertation Abstracts International, 56*(3-A), 874.

Skjerve, J., Nielsen, G. H., Jacobsen, C. H., Gullestad, S. E., Hansen, B. R., Reichelt, S., & Torgersen, A. M. (2009). Nondisclosure in psychotherapy group supervision: The supervisor perspective. *Nordic Psychology, 61*(4), 28–48.

Sobell, L. C., Manor, H. L., Sobell, M. B., & Dum, M. (2008). Self-critiques of audiotaped therapy sessions: A motivational procedure for facilitating feedback during supervision. *Training and Education in Professional Psychology, 2*(3), 151–155.

Sommer, C. A., & Cox, J. A. (2003). Using Greek mythology as a metaphor to enhance supervision. *Counselor Education and Supervision, 42*(4), 326–336.

Son, E., Ellis, M. V., & Yoo, S.-K. (2013). Clinical supervision in South Korea and the United States: A comparative descriptive study. *The Counseling Psychologist, 41*(1), 48–65.

Sorlie, T., Gammon, D., Bergvik, S., & Sexton, H. (1999). Psychotherapy supervision face-to-face and by video conferencing: A comparative study. *British Journal of Psychotherapy, 15*(4), 452–462.

Stoltenberg, C. D. (1981). Approaching supervision from a developmental perspective: The counselor complexity model. *Journal of Counseling Psychology, 28*(1), 59–65.

Stoltenberg, C. D., Bailey, K. C., Cruzan, C. B., Hart, J. T., & Ukuku, U. (2014). The integrative developmental model of supervision. In C. E. Watkins & D. L. Milne (Eds.), *The Wiley International Handbook of Clinical Supervision* (pp. 576–597). Chichester, UK: Wiley Blackwell.

Stoltenberg, C. D., & McNeill, B. W. (2010). *IDM supervision: An integrative developmental model for supervising counselors and therapists* (3rd ed.). New York: Routledge.

Stoltenberg, C. D., McNeill, B., & Delworth, U. (1998). *IDM: The integrated developmental model of clinical supervision.* San Francisco: Jossey-Bass.

Sue, D., & Sue, D. W. (2008). *Counseling the culturally diverse: Theory and practice.* Hoboken, NJ: Wiley.

Sue, D. W., Arredondo, P., & McDavis, R. J. (1992). Multicultural counseling competencies and standards: A call to the profession. *Journal of Counseling and Development, 70*(4), 477–486.

Sussman, T., Bogo, M., & Globerman, J. (2007). Field instructor perceptions in group supervision: Establishing trust through managing group dynamics. *The Clinical Supervisior, 26*(1–2), 61–80.

Swift, J. K., Callahan, J. L., Rousmaniere, T. G., Whipple, J. L., Dexter, K., & Wrape, E. R. (2014). Using client outcome monitoring as a tool for supervision. *Psychotherapy, 52*(2), 180–184.

Tangen, J. L., & Borders, D. (2016). The supervisory relationship: A conceptual and psychometric review of measures. *Counselor Education and Supervision, 55,* 159–181.

Tervalon, M., & Murray-Garcia, J. (1998). Cultural humility versus cultural competence: A critical distinction in defining physician training outcomes in multicultural education. *Journal of Health Care for the Poor and Underserved, 9*(2), 117–125.

Thomas, J. T. (2007). Informed consent through contracting for supervision: Minimizing risks, enhancing benefits. *Professional Psychology: Research and Practice, 38*(3), 221–231.

Thomas, J. T. (2010). *Ethical and legal issues in supervision and consultation.* Washington, DC: American Psychological Association.

Thomas, J. T. (2014). International ethics for psychotherapy supervisors: Principles, practices and future directions. In C. E. Watkins & D. L. Milne (Eds.), *The Wiley International Handbook of Clinical Supervision* (pp. 131–154). Chichester, UK: Wiley Blackwell.

Tracey, T. J., Bludworth, J., & Glidden-Tracey, C. E. (2012). Are there parallel processes in psychotherapy supervision? An empirical examination. *Psychotherapy, 49*(3), 330–343.

Tracey, T. J., Ellickson, J. L., & Sherry, P. (1989). Reactance in relation to different supervisory environments and counselor development. *Journal of Counseling Psychology, 36*(3), 336–344.

Tsui, M. S., O'Donoghue, K., & Ng, A. K. (2014). Culturally competent and diversity-sensitive clinical supervision. In C. E. Watkins & D. L. Milne (Eds.), *The Wiley International Handbook of Clinical Supervision* (pp. 238–254). Chichester, UK: Wiley Blackwell.

Tuckman, B. W. (1965). Developmental sequence in small groups. *Psychological Bulletin, 63*(6), 384–399.

Tuckman, B. W., & Jensen, M. A. C. (1977). Stages of small-group development revisited. *Group & Organization Management, 2*(4), 419–427.

Turpin, G., & Wheeler, S. (2011). IAPT supervision guidance (revised March 2011). Retrieved from http://www.iapt.nhs.uk/silo/files/iapt-supervision-guidance-revised-march-2011.pdf

Valadez, A. A., & Garcia, J. L. (1998). In a different light: An environmental metaphor of counselor supervision. *Journal of Professional Counseling, Practice, Theory, & Research, 26*(2), 92–106.

Vargas, L. A., Porter, N., & Falender, C. A. (2008). Supervision, culture, and context. In C. A. Falender & E. P. Shafranske (Eds.), *Casebook for clinical supervision: A competency-based approach* (pp. 121–136). Washington, DC: American Psychological Association.

Vassilas, C., & Ho, L. (2000). Video for teaching purposes. *Advances in Psychiatric Treatment, 6*(4), 304–311.

Veach, P. M. (2001). Conflict and counterproductivity in supervision—when relationships are less than ideal: Comment on Nelson and Friedlander (2001) and Gray et al. (2001). *Journal of Counseling Psychology, 48*(4), 396–400.

Vespia, K. M., Heckman-Stone, C., & Delworth, U. (2002). Describing and facilitating effective supervision behavior in counseling trainees. *Psychotherapy: Theory, Research, Practice, Training, 39*(1), 56–65.

Vincent, C. (2010). *The essentials of patient safety*. Hoboken, NJ: Wiley-Blackwell.

Vygotsky, L. S. (1978). *Mind in society: The development of higher mental processes*. Cambridge, MA: Harvard University Press.

Wainwright, N. A. (2010). *The development of the Leeds Alliance in Supervision Scale (LASS): A brief sessional measure of the supervisory alliance*. Unpublished DClinPsych thesis, University of Leeds, UK.

Warner, P. (1998). *The role of perceived gender-related personality traits in initial supervisory relationships*. Unpublished doctoral dissertation, University of Missouri. *Dissertation Abstracts International, 60* (4-B), 1904.

Watkins, C. E. (1995). Pathological attachment styles in psychotherapy supervision. *Psychotherapy: Theory, Research, Practice, Training, 32*(2), 333–340.

Watkins, C. E. (1997). *Handbook of psychotherapy supervision*. New York: Wiley.

Watkins, C. E. (2010). Psychoanalytic constructs in psychotherapy supervision. *American Journal of Psychotherapy, 64*(4), 393–416.

Watkins, C. E. (2011a). Does psychotherapy supervision contribute to patient outcomes? Considering thirty years of research. *The Clinical Supervisor, 30*(2), 235–256.

Watkins, C. E. (2011b). The real relationship in psychotherapy supervision. *American Journal of Psychotherapy, 65*, 99–116.

Watkins, C. E. (2014a). The supervisory alliance: A half century of theory, practice, and research in critical perspective. *American Journal of Psychotherapy, 68*(1), 19–55.

Watkins, C. E. (2014b). The supervisory alliance as quintessential integrative variable. *Journal of Contemporary Psychotherapy, 44*, 151–161.

Watkins, C. E., & Hook, J. N. (2016). On a culturally humble psychoanalytic supervision perspective: Creating the cultural third. *Psychoanalytic Psychology, 33*(3), 487–517.

Watkins, C. E., & Milne, D. (Eds.) (2014). *The Wiley International Handbook of Clinical Supervision*. Chichester, UK: Wiley Blackwell.

Watkins, C. E., & Riggs, S. A. (2012). Psychotherapy supervision and attachment theory: Review, reflections, and recommendations. *The Clinical Supervisor, 31*(2), 256–289.

Weingardt, K. R., Cucciare, M. A., Bellotti, C., & Lai, W. P. (2009). A randomized trial comparing two models of web-based training in cognitive-behavioral therapy for substance abuse counselors. *Journal of Substance Abuse Treatment, 37*(3), 219–227.

Wheeler, S., Aveline, M., & Barkham, M. (2011). Practice-based supervision research: A network of researchers using a common toolkit. *Counselling and Psychotherapy Research, 11*(2), 88–96.

Wheeler, S., & Richards, K. (2007). The impact of clinical supervision on counsellors and therapists, their practice and their clients: A systematic review of the literature. *Counselling and Psychotherapy Research, 7*(1), 54–65.

White, E., & Winstanley, J. (2010). A randomised controlled trial of clinical supervision: selected findings from a novel Australian attempt to establish the evidence base for causal relationships with quality of care and patient outcomes, as an informed contribution to mental health nursing practice development. *Journal of Research in Nursing, 15*(2), 151–167.

White, V. E., & Queener, J. (2003). Supervisor and supervisee attachments and social provisions related to the supervisory working alliance. *Counselor Education and Supervision, 42*(3), 203–218.

White, M. B., & Russell, C. S. (1997). Examining the multifaceted notion of isomorphism in marriage and family therapy supervision: A quest for conceptual clarity. *Journal of Marital and Family Therapy, 23*(3), 315–333.

Whittaker, S. M. (2004). *A multi-vocal synthesis of supervisees' anxiety and self-efficacy during clinical supervision: Meta-analysis and interviews.* Unpublished doctoral dissertion, Virginia Polytechnic Institute and State University.

Wiggins, G. P. (1998). *Educative assessment: Designing assessments to inform and improve student performance* (Vol. 1). San Francisco: Jossey-Bass.

Wood, B. P. (2000). Feedback: A key feature of medical training 1. *Radiology, 215*(1), 17–19.

Woodbridge, K., & Fulford, B. (2004). *Whose values? A workbook for values-based practice in mental health care.* London: Sainsbury Centre for Mental Health.

Woodward, H. (1998). Reflective journals and portfolios: Learning through assessment. *Assessment and Evaluation in higher Education, 23*(4), 415–423.

Worthen, V. E., & Lambert, M. J. (2007). Outcome oriented supervision: Advantages of adding systematic client tracking to supportive consultations. *Counselling and Psychotherapy Research, 7*(1), 48–53.

Worthen, V., & McNeill, B. W. (1996). A phenomenological investigation of "good" supervision events. *Journal of Counseling Psychology, 43*(1), 25–34.

Worthen, V. E., & McNeill, B. W. (1996). A phenomenological investigation of "good" supervision events. *Journal of Counseling Psychology, 43*(1), 25–34.

Worthington, E. L. (1984). Use of trait labels in counseling supervision by experienced and inexperienced supervisors. *Professional Psychology: Research and Practice, 15*(3), 457–461.

Worthington, E. L., & Stern, A. (1985). Effects of supervisor and supervisee degree level and gender on the supervisory relationship. *Journal of Counseling Psychology, 32*(2), 252–262.

Wrape, E. R., Callahan, J. L., Ruggero, C. J., & Watkins, C. E. (2015). An exploration of faculty supervisor variables and their impact on client outcomes. *Training and Education in Professional Psychology, 9*(1), 35–43.

Xavier, K., Shepherd, L., & Goldstein, D. (2007). Clinical supervision and education via videoconference: A feasibility project. *Journal of Telemedicine and Telecare, 13*(4), 206–209.

Yourman, D. B. (2003). Trainee disclosure in psychotherapy supervision: The impact of shame. *Journal of Clinical Psychology, 59*(5), 601–609.

Index

Please note that 'SR' stands for 'supervisory relationship', whenever it appears. Page references to Boxes, Figures and Tables are in *italics*, followed by the letters '*b*', '*f*', or '*t*', as appropriate.

Effective Supervisory Relationships: Best Evidence and Practice, First Edition.
Helen Beinart and Sue Clohessy.
© 2017 John Wiley & Sons Ltd. Published 2017 by John Wiley & Sons Ltd.